MW00606376

Praise for
The Healthy Conscious Traveler

It takes a traveler to advise a traveler, and Robyn Benson is magnificently qualified to do so. Moreover, she is one of the outstanding experts in integrative medicine in the U.S., and she has spread her wisdom worldwide. Modern travel is increasingly complex and demanding. It can be either uplifting or a downer and a hazard to your health. To make sure your travel adds to your life, read Benson's fine book.

> Larry Dossey, M.D., author of *Reinventing Medicine* and *The Power of Premonitions*

I travel more than 150 days per year. Over the last few years, I have been free from jet lag, fatigue, and other post-flight symptoms. Why? In 2009 I was blessed to meet Dr. Robyn Benson! Robyn is a gifted healer and a passionate champion for wellness. This book is filled with her wise and practical advice. It will guide you to become a healthy conscious traveler.

> Michael J. Gelb, author of *How to Think Like Leonardo Da Vinci* and *Brain Power: Improve Your Mind as You Age*

Even those who do not fly around the world often travel 10,000 miles or more each year in automobiles. Let your favorite form of travel sustain you with the true health solutions Robyn provides.

> C. Norman Shealy, M.D., Ph.D., author of *Living Bliss* and *Life beyond 100*

As both an exceptionally skilled and inventive practitioner of natural medicine and a passionate traveler, Dr. Robyn Benson has managed to visit 70 countries in her 50 years, while treating 80,000 patients at her clinic and never experiencing a sick day off in over 23 years of practice. How? In this indispensable and wise book, Dr. Benson shares a bouquet of intensely practical tips, along with other practices, technologies, common sense, and wisdom that support your thriving vitality. At home and on the road, don't leave home without The Healthy Conscious Traveler.

Kenny Ausubel, Co-CEO and founder (in 1990) of "Bioneers," and an award-winning social entrepreneur, journalist, author and filmmaker

A must-read for every traveler who has ever suffered through stress and sickness while on the road — so essentially, everyone. This book will always *be on my packing list!*

Hyla Cass M.D., author of *8 Weeks to Vibrant Health* and *Supplement Your Prescription: What Your Doctor Doesn't Know About Nutrition*

With The Healthy Conscious Traveler, *Dr. Robyn Benson has put together a very important book that outlines in great detail all the perils of travel* and *offers practical, user-friendly solutions. I have experienced many of the issues Robyn discusses in my time as a military and commercial airline pilot. With a friendly, inviting tone and simple explanations for complicated topics, she is an engaging companion as she shares critical information that will transform your life.*

John Cote, Founder of Healthcare Elsewhere, the world's leading medical tourism show

Whether you travel near or far, frequently or occasionally, Dr. Robyn Benson's groundbreaking The Healthy Conscious Traveler *provides essential guidelines as well as inspiration for safe, healthy travel from a seasoned health care provider and a veteran adventure traveler. If you have not read this book, you are not ready for your next trip!*

Dr. Nalini Chilkov, Founder, www.integrativecanceranswers.com/

Dr. Robyn Benson's life-long passion for both travel and natural medicine has come to fruition in her leading-edge book The Healthy Conscious Traveler. *A must read for any traveler, she shares attainable and thought provoking guidelines how to maintain and optimize your* health while traveling for business or vacation. From enjoyable and attainable self-care practices to advanced technology that provide solutions, Dr. Benson will reveal her secrets to know how to stay healthy in a world flooded with toxic chemicals, food and energy sources. The information in The Healthy Conscious Traveler is vital for anyone, not just travelers interested in overall better health.

Jan Kinder, RN, HN-BC, CMT

The Healthy Conscious Traveler is a groundbreaking book by a true thought leader that will change the life of every traveler! It's packed with great information on how to stay healthy, happy and have fun while you travel, **all** written in a user-friendly way. Don't take off for your next trip without this!

Marcia Wieder, CEO/Founder, Dream University

Ironically, I can wear out my health by traveling up to nine months a year to speak to groups about how to maintain health. While I certainly know to avoid eating genetically engineered foods (that's my topic), there's lots of additional healthy traveling tips I've never heard of. So I could theoretically take a year off and collect all the cutting edge theories that would help me stay healthy while on the road, or I can simply read Robyn's book. The choice is obvious. (I'll read it on the plane.)

Jeffrey M. Smith - Director of the award-winning film, Genetic Roulette – The Gamble of Our Lives

I highly recommend this book! Dr. Robyn Benson tackles head-on the GMO concerns of travelers, as well as the dangers of toxic jet fuels, radiation, parasites, motion sickness and so much more. She does not miss a beat, offering an impressive array of solutions for traveling safely, allergy-free, and staying healthy for your next fun filled adventure. The Healthy Conscious Traveler will completely change the way you travel as well as change your life!

Dr. Susanne Bennett, bestselling author of The 7-Day Allergy Makeover and host of the Wellness for Life show on RadioMD & iHeart Radio

In The Healthy Conscious Traveler, *Dr. Robyn Benson shows you how to protect your immune system, increase your energy, renew vigor and stamina—all while traveling the world with superb health. She is the best kind of doctor, cutting edge and thoughtful. Her approach allows you to incorporate tips and strategies into your daily life so that you can start to look and feel fantastic.*

I highly recommend this book for anyone who travels short or long distances. Most of what Dr. Robyn Benson teaches you can be done on your own, empowering you to be in control of your health for the rest of your life. Read this book and become a Healthy Conscious Traveler!

Dr. Marcella Vonn Harting, Ph.D,.
bestselling author of *Yes, No, Maybe*
Chronobiotic Nutrition, Guerrilla
Multilevel Marketing

The Healthy Conscious Traveler *is not only a must-read, it is a must-refer-to trusted travel companion. Dr. Robyn Benson has skillfully woven a lifetime of global travel experiences with her extensive medical expertise to discuss known and invisible influences impacting our health. What you have is a guide filled with cutting-edge information, innovative solutions and the best practices to sustain your greatest health as you travel—in life, wherever you go.*

Dr. Joan Rosenberg, Psychologist, creator
of Emotional Mastery Training and host
of the *Mindstream* podcast

THE HEALTHY
CONSCIOUS TRAVELER

8 Pathways to Smart and Effortless Travel

Robyn Benson, D.O.M.

Santa Fe, NM

The Healthy Conscious Traveler:
8 Pathways to Smart and Effortless Travel
by Robyn Benson, D.O.M.

ISBN-13: 978-0-9962781-1-9 (color paperback)

ISBN-13: 978-0-9962781-3-3 (b/w paperback)

ISBN-13: 978-0-9962781-4-0 (ebook: Kindle / mobi)

ISBN-13: 978-0-9962781-0-2 (ebook: epub)

Find out more at www.robynbenson.com

Printed in the United States

I am dedicating this book to the "change agents" and the "way seers" of the world who are pioneering new and better ways to "travel" through life, while honoring Mother Earth foremost and our physical embodiment of her.

The Grace of Travel

By Robyn Benson

I am grateful for the man who moved his seat so my young daughter could sit next to me,

and for the lady who put her wrinkled hand on mine when I was scared during turbulence,

and for the stranger who sat next to me and became my lifelong friend,

for the humor of the flight attendant who made a sold-out, five hour delayed flight fun,

for the pilot who course-directed for our safety, for my tethered passport with 60 country stamps,

for travel delays that saved our lives due to inclement weather, and for trips that carried me across the world in fewer than 24 hours,

for the man who helped me lift my luggage twice,

for the sweet young girl who let me use her cell phone when I lost mine,

for the Call to Prayer in Egypt and flying over voluptuous clouds, for the wonders of the world that have changed my life,

for healing my sense of separation and opening me to unity in diversity

and for the chance to see wild animals roaming freely in Kenya,

and for journeying the footsteps of the Buddha in India, and walking the stations of Christ's last day in Israel.

Contents

The Healthy Conscious Traveler's Resources
from www.robynbenson.com

* *Healthy Conscious Traveler's Food Guide*

* *Healthy Conscious Traveler's First-Aid Kit*

Foreword

Traveling can be one of life's greatest pleasures. And it also provides a special opportunity for us to expand consciousness. As
philosopher Martin Buber explains, "All journeys have secret destinations of which the traveler is unaware."

Mark Twain elaborates: "Travel is fatal to prejudice, bigotry and
narrow-mindedness and many of our people need it sorely on these
accounts. Broad, wholesome, charitable views of men and things cannot be acquired by vegetating in one little corner of the earth all one's
lifetime." There's no better way to expand one's understanding of self
and the world than to explore different lands, cultures and customs.

I love to travel. And that's a good thing, because since 1980,
I've averaged about 150 days on the road each year. In the last 12
months, I've been to Italy three times, to Turkey, Ireland, London,
Holland and Mexico and back and forth across the U.S. It sounds
glamorous and sometimes it is, but other times it's exhausting. In
any case, I need to stay healthy and keep my energy up, because
when I arrive at my destination, I usually must give a keynote
speech and a workshop the next day.

How do I stay healthy? (The last time I had a cold was seven years
ago.) How do I maintain my energy level? (I've never missed an engage-
ment in 35 years and I love what I do more than ever.) In other words,
how do I avoid looking like my passport photo? All of my strategies are
presented here, in *The Healthy Conscious Traveler* by Dr. Robyn Benson.

Upon returning from a trip, the first appointment I schedule is
with Dr. Benson for an acupuncture tune-up and electromagnetic
balancing session. If this isn't geographically possible for you, don't
worry, because thanks to this book, you can bring her wisdom and
healing energy with you wherever you go.

Dr. Benson is the pioneer of a global movement for health em-
powerment she calls "The Self-care Revolution" and in this revolutionary book she guides you to care for yourself when you must face
the stresses of travel. And those stresses are greater than ever before.

This book is filled with useful, practical tips for self-care, most of
which are applicable and important even if you never leave your home.
And Dr. Benson does a superb job of elucidating the special challenges
and stresses that we face when we head for the airport. The advice she

offers isn't just from her perspective as an experienced clinician and healer but also as someone who travels frequently herself.

She is particularly passionate about sharing her insight into becoming a "Frequency Flier." She explains that frequent travel can have a deleterious effect on your bio-frequency, thereby weakening your immune system and making you more susceptible to a range of ailments. This is why many people experience fatigue and exhaustion after flying, even if they follow wise advice on diet, exercise, etc. Bio-frequency is one of the "missing links" in most guides to healthy travel. Dr. Benson is an expert in this area and she offers a number of simple strategies for adjusting and balancing your energy when you're on the road.

Dr. Benson references Gregory Bateson, anthropologist and author of *Steps to an Ecology of Mind*, who wrote: "The major problems in the world are the result of the difference between the way nature works and the way people think." In *The Healthy Conscious Traveler*, Dr. Benson devotes her wisdom, developed over more than 23 years of practice as a Doctor of Oriental Medicine, to help us bridge the gap between our habits of mind and the workings of nature.

Dr. Benson helps us cultivate habits of mind that are more harmonious with the workings of nature both externally and internally. She emphasizes the role that attitude, consciousness and intention play in our wellness at all times, but especially when we travel. Your body/mind system is a remarkably potent pharmacy and the best medicine is that which you generate yourself. She offers wonderful insights on how to maintain perspective and alignment with deeper purpose in the face of travel challenges such as airport delays and flight turbulence. If you are stranded in an airport for 11 hours due to weather or "mechanical problems," Dr. Benson will show you how to avoid "terminal illness."

Author Henry Miller wrote: "One's destination is never a place but a new way of seeing things." *The Healthy Conscious Traveler* offers a new perspective on self-care, so you can arrive at all your destinations with more awareness, energy and delight.

Michael J. Gelb
Author of *How to Think Like Leonardo da Vinci* and *Creativity on Demand*

Santa Fe, New Mexico
May 2015

Introduction: Becoming a Healthy Conscious Traveler

All journeys have secret destinations of which the traveler is unaware. ~ Martin Buber

Are You Ready to Be an Energized, Fit and Conscious Traveler?

Do you spend a significant portion of your life in planes, trains or automobiles? If so, you've probably noticed that every means of transportation has become busier and more crowded than ever. The travel industry has changed immensely since the advent of commercial air travel in the 1920s. Airlines have cut back flights with the aim of packing smaller planes to capacity, and traffic, whether in the air or on the road, is more congested than ever before. Meanwhile, long-distance travel has become an integral part of our personal and professional lifestyles.

Travel can be one of life's greatest adventures, but for many people it has become more than just a hassle; it has become a threat to their health and well-being. The nature of this threat goes beyond just the stress associated with Homeland Security pat downs and road rage. In addition to these obvious stressors, travel stress has a hidden dimension: airplanes, cars, buses and trains all emit unhealthy electromagnetic frequencies.

I regularly see patients who are frequent travelers, and I also have a number of clients who are flight attendants and pilots. They come to my office suffering from exhaustion and a range of chronic illnesses. Many of them spend more than 30 hours a week in airports, airplanes and cars. This kind of travel tremendously exhausts all of the body's systems, especially the nervous, digestive, hormone and immune systems.

Recently I was watching television and waiting for my flight at the gate in the St. Louis airport while the president was delivering the State of the Union address. He boasted that the U.S. has the best, most advanced transportation system in the world. He also defended his Affordable Health Care legislation. As a health practitioner, I support all efforts to make healthcare more accessible and affordable, but there was a missing element in the president's remarks. Our relatively efficient travel system also exposes us, unknowingly, to high levels of radiation and other pollution on a daily basis. It is essential to raise awareness within this industry in order to reduce the exponential growth of related chronic health problems. We can reduce healthcare costs and improve the quality of life for everyone who travels by practicing the simple approaches I will introduce in this book.

As a seasoned world traveler and Doctor of Oriental Medicine who's been practicing for more than two decades, I have gained great insight into how travel impacts the physiology of the body. I've witnessed the effects of travel-related stress on my patients and sought ways to help them recover. More importantly, I've focused on educating my patients so that they can better protect themselves from the debilitating effects of the artificial environments through which they move. As a frequent traveler myself, I have a passionate interest in studying the best ways to protect you from the fatigue and disease-inducing effects of contemporary technology.

If you've ever lost the first few days of your vacation recovering from travel fatigue, or if you suffer from serious jet lag or a tendency to get a sore throat or sinus infection after a flight, then you are probably being affected by the artificial electromagnetic fields, airborne microbes and other toxins. This travel-related assault on your body is foremost from high levels of distorting frequencies that emanate from Wi-Fi, cell phones, computers, routers, server rooms, cell towers, cordless phones and plasma screens.

If you are on your umpteenth business trip of the year and are feeling run-down and unsatisfied with the quality of your life; if travel is now equated with stress and depression and you are "wired and tired"; and if, like many of my patients, you have thought to yourself, "Traveling is too tiring and is such a hassle, I would rather stay home," then, this book is for you!

In 1886, the great genius of electromagnetic research Nikola Tesla said that the advent of electricity and artificial currencies would be both a blessing and a curse to all of life. My intention is to show you how to protect yourself from the curse so you can take advantage of the blessings.

We all know that when driving, red means stop, green means go and yellow means proceed with caution. Likewise, with your health while traveling or at home, we can use a similar system to stop accidents, disease and stress. Green might not always be available to you, but even getting from red to yellow can save you a lot of pain and discomfort. We will refer back to green, yellow and red often in this book, and it's important enough that you might want to copy this schematic and keep it in your wallet or purse to reference when you travel.

Take a look at the Red Zone of "Electrified Times" in Figure A. The Red Zone reveals the unhealthy frequencies (60-1,600+ Hz) that we are living with more than ever each day. If you live in this Red Zone for too long, your body begins to break down. The Yellow Zone (30-60 Hz) is the warning zone where many of us live. Our bodies are giving us signs of stress, our hormones are all over the place and our brains are not functioning optimally. The Green Zone (0-30 Hz) is where we thrive and survive on a cellular level. This is what we all must strive for by following The 8 Pathways in this book. This is ultimately the thriving zone where illness does not exist.

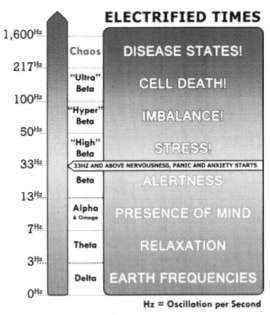

Figure A

Soon, we will introduce the Ultimate Health Plan that will show you step by step how to keep your mind and body healthy as easily as you drive your car to avoid accidents.

I imagine that you are opening this book with a sincere interest in solving the many health-related travel issues we all face. I'll bet you would like to know that it is possible to travel and still feel great and to return from your travel rejuvenated, rested and full of beautiful memories. Yes, this is possible and more! No need to cancel your future trips or put your suitcases away forever.

You can become what I call a Healthy Conscious Traveler (HCT)

I have a love affair with travel, especially when I go to new corners of the world and experience unfamiliar sights, sounds, scents and cultural ways that provide a feast for my soul. I travel often to recharge from my busy work life. Whether I travel alone, with a friend or in a group, it has always been a goal of mine to leave with a healthy immune system, while preparing for the possible headache, blister, sinus infection or food poisoning. I'm committed to my positive lifestyle habits while away, and my goal is to return home healthy and ready to dive back into my life. After more than 23 years of significant travel, I have never missed a day of work, thanks to the practices I will share with you in these pages.

As you navigate through this book, I hope that you will not only cultivate the mindset of healthy traveling but you will also see yourself as a Healthy Conscious Traveler, which is how I will refer to you throughout this book. As an HCT, you will learn to be more aware of your body, thoughts, reactions and surroundings. You will prepare your immune system during the days or even weeks ahead of your trip. *You will become a personally empowered individual who knows that your health is in your own hands, not just your doctor's hands.*

As the CEO of your own wellness, you will know that you only get sick when your immune system is low due to stress, poor dietary habits and other choices that compromise your resistance. You'll know that the coughing child, who inevitably sits behind you in the airplane, or the man next to you in the security line who sneezes loudly without using a handkerchief isn't the cause of your illness. Rather, it's the internal state of your immune system.

As a Healthy Conscious Traveler, you will learn to follow The 8 Pathways to strengthen your immune system and experience great health when you are on the road, as well as when you return home. You'll retrain, regain and renew yourself for travel success by following the program outlined here.

THE 8 PATHWAYS

1. **Be your own best health-care advocate.**

2. **Reconnect to the earth regularly.**

3. **Eat natural, organic food.**

4. **Drink lots of pure water.**

5. **Stay active.**

6. **Optimize sleep.**

7. **Stay conscious and travel with intention and stress resiliency.**

8. **Connect regularly to your higher self through mindful techniques.**

As an HCT, you know the value of everyday wellness and understand that health is a way of life, not a matter of luck or good genes. As you develop the confidence to make positive health changes and embody the messages in this book, the ripple of your choices will change the quality, attitude and longevity of your life. My experience is that greater vitality and radiant health always translate into deeper happiness.

On a 48-hour plane trip to Bhutan, I was reading the book, *The Geography of Bliss, One Grump's Search for the Happiest Places in the World* by Eric Weiner. According to Weiner, Bhutan is one of the happiest places in the world, and I felt truly blessed to have had the opportunity to travel there and experience its emotional richness for myself.

But what makes Bhutan a happy country? Bhutan is often referred to as a "living culture" because its residents realize their connectedness to nature and all of life. Bhutan's living culture makes it one of the most progressive and sustainable countries in the world. Its residents revere the earth and the quality of their healthy environment. Bhutan is the ideal microcosm of the potential that any country has to catalyze a healthier and restorative existence. Discovering healthy lifestyles has been part of my quest while traveling, so being part of this culture was a happy and memorable time for me.

How different would the world be if more countries adopted this reverence for life, rather than the primary reverence for money or power? How can we learn from Bhutan and apply the principles of this living, healthy culture to all industries, especially the travel industry?

I have had the great fortune to travel to more than 70 countries in my 50 years of life. I vividly remember flying from Syracuse, New York, to Washington, DC, for the first time when I was 16, soaring above the clouds at 30,000 feet, reading and talking to nearby passengers. I loved the feeling of freedom and I quickly became a travel aficionado. I was also grateful for all of my previous car, bus and train rides. A seed had been planted, and I was ready to see the whole world. I had not only found my passion but also experienced a deep love for seeing the world and connecting with all of its people, cultures and traditions. I began to understand more fully what it is that connects us all.

I believe this universal connection is beyond our primary needs of water, food and air. In my opinion, it is our traditions, our history and our most basic need of being touched and expressing and receiving love. We need each other. I found this to be most evident among the Masai tribal people in Kenya. Their need for food and water directs them to their next habitation, but as they travel, they celebrate. Their vibrantly colored headdresses and jewelry are part of everyday life and reflect the joy that they feel each day. They come alive as they sing songs praising and honoring Mother Earth and expressing deep gratitude for everything the earth provides. They realize their life depends completely on their relationship with each other, the earth, the sun, the sky, fire, water, air and the infinite cosmos, and they are simply and beautifully happy.

My journey to Bhutan, as well as time spent with the Masai and other indigenous people of the world, has made me more aware of the fact that breathing fresh air, walking barefoot on the earth and nourishing ourselves with whole foods is integral to the formula for healthy traveling. This is the ultimate in healthy living, which is essential for sustaining our future generations.

As I'm writing *The Healthy Conscious Traveler,* we are witnessing tremendous shifts in our consciousness as individuals with the purpose to connect with each other through grassroots activism and on the Internet. The movement has begun and we find ourselves at the very tipping point of immense change. We are witnessing massive global efforts to make this world a better place in terms of new energy, vibrant health and monetary and educational options.

My aim is to guide you in the discovery of how you can adopt the wisdom of the Bhutanese, the Masai and other indigenous peoples I've met and apply it to our contemporary, complex world.

Valuable travel facts for the HCT to be aware of: statistics and facts on the global tourism industry

According to the website The Statistics Portal, the travel and tourism industry is one of the world's largest industries, with a global economic contribution of almost $7 trillion in 2013. The direct economic impact of the industry, including accommodation, transportation, entertainment and attractions, was approximately $2.2 trillion that year. A number of countries, including France and the U.S., are consistently popular tourism destinations, but other, less well-known countries are quickly emerging in order to reap the economic benefits of the industry.

Worldwide, the tourism industry has experienced steady growth almost every year. International tourist arrivals increased from 528 million in 2005 to 1.09 billion in 2013. Figures are forecasted to exceed 1.8 billion by 2030. Each year, Europe receives the most international tourist arrivals. It also produces the most travelers: with just fewer than 566 million outbound tourists in 2013, the region had more than double that of the second largest tourist origin, the Asia-Pacific region.

In 2013, global international tourism revenue reached approximately $1.16 trillion, having almost doubled since 2005. That same year, China had the largest international tourism expenditure, followed by the U.S. and Germany. The leading city in international visitor spending was London, where tourists spent more than $19 billion in 2014.

FACTS ABOUT THE GLOBAL TOURISM INDUSTRY
(FROM THE STATISTICS PORTAL)

Global Tourism Overview	Values
Total contribution of travel & tourism to global economy	$6,990.3bn
Number of international tourist arrivals worldwide	1,087m
Number of European tourist arrivals	563.4m
International Tourist Expenditure	
Global international tourism revenue	$1,159bn
International tourism expenditure of the United States	$86.2bn
China's market share of tourism expenditure	11.1%
Lodging and Accommodation	
Global hotel industry total revenue	$457bn
Average price of a hotel room in Europe	$185
Average price of a hotel room in North America	$119
Daily hotel rate in New York	$309.86
Online Travel Market	
Percentage of travel bookings made from the U.S.	39%
Online travel bookings revenue worldwide	$340bn
Online travel agencies' share of total hotel industry revenue in the U.S.	8.4%
Cruise Industry	
Market volume of the cruise industry in North America	$17.46bn
Revenue of the cruise industry worldwide	$39.6bn
Average cruise revenue per passenger worldwide	$1728

The website TheRichest.com has found that the direct economic impact of the travel and tourism industry, at $2.2 trillion, is twice that of the alcohol industry—the richest (legal) industry in the world at the same time. And the indirect economic impact of travel and tourism, at $7 trillion, is greater than the total of the top 10 richest industries and companies in the world.(1)

1	Alcohol Industry	$1,161 billion
2	OPEC Revenue	$1,027 billion
3	Global Pharma Market	$950 billion
4	Apple	$500 billion
5	Worldwide TV Industry	$364 billion
6	Walmart	$228 billion
7	Microsoft	$224 billion
8	Google	$187 billion
9	EBay	$175 billion
10	BP	$132 billion
	TOTAL	$4,948 billion

As you read these travel facts from Air Transport Action Group website(2) and reflect on your own traveling history, consider how knowing this information may inspire you to make healthy choices not only with travel but, more importantly, as a way of life, each and every day.

- In 2010, 33 million people were employed worldwide in aviation and tourism.

- In 2010, 649 million tons of CO_2 were produced from worldwide flights.

- 1,715 airlines (including small regional ones) operate a fleet of 23,000 aircraft serving 3,750 airports through a route network of several million kilometers managed by 160 air navigation service providers

- The aviation industry generates $425 billion of GDP per year and consumes 1.5 billion barrels of fuel annually.

- Flight and Radiation Exposure Fact: The average flight across the U.S. emits 3-5 mrem, which is approximately equivalent to one chest X-ray.(3)

- Due to cost, oxygen is not offered during flights, but what *is* offered is circulated air, which provides the perfect environment for harboring viruses and germs.(4)

- Blood oxygen saturation during commercial flights can be 5 to10% lower than normal. If you are healthy, this low saturation level shouldn't be a problem. However, if you have any medical conditions, you must consult your physician.(5)

- Airlines mishandle more than 20 million bags a year and can take up to a week or more to match the bag to its owner. Also, every 3.5 seconds, someone in America loses a cell phone. Most found items are not returned because the finder cannot easily locate the owner.(6)

Imagine if the travel industry was a leader in creating a healthy future by providing an electro-smog and pollution-free environments, as well as providing proper care to their flight crews and travelers. Each and every pilot and flight attendant I interviewed said this was a high priority for them. Whether they have worked in the field for one year or 35, they found that the health aspects and possible hazards of their jobs were mostly ignored. This book offers ideas and solutions to catalyze the traveling industry into creating a healthy work and travel environment.

But don't fret. You are an HCT, a Healthy Conscious Traveler. In *The Healthy Conscious Traveler*, you will discover the importance of a healthy diet, ideal water consumption, effective exercise and the best and most critical ways to prepare and support your body for your traveling journey. You will further understand the difference between healthy and unhealthy frequencies and why your entire well-being is dependent on a healthy electrical system around and in your body. This book also includes assessment tools to rate your level of sensitivity.

This is the beginning of your journey as a Healthy Conscious Traveler. I am grateful to guide and inspire you along the way. *Bon Voyage!*

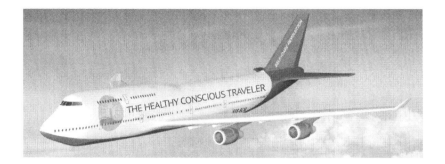

Chapter 1

Are You a *Frequency* Flier?

*The greatest medical advances of the next decade will come
from manipulating the body's flow of energy.
~ Dr. Mehmet Oz*

I have titled this chapter, "Are You a *Frequency* Flier?" because as
you "fly" from one form of transportation to another, you are moving in thousands of different frequencies. Be informed that unless
you live deep in the wilderness, Wi-Fi and smart meter frequencies
from neighbors' homes, nearby stores and office buildings are traveling through your home at this very moment.

As you pack for your next trip, I am sure you won't forget your
prescription drugs. Are you perhaps taking a prescription remedy
for one of these travel-related health challenges, including sleeplessness, anxiety, dizziness, palpitations, depression, ADHD, headaches or gastrointestinal distress?

What about your young children? Are they being treated with
pharmaceutical drugs for any of the above symptoms? If so, have
you ever considered that all the artificial frequencies that surround
you, including Wi-Fi, cell phones and cell phone towers, smart meters, high voltage electrical lines and such, may be the actual cause
of some of their problems? I see this often in my practice with
hundreds of patients. It is difficult to escape from these harmful

frequencies, HCT, so read carefully as I share some important information that even your doctor may not know about.

A young woman came to see me with every single symptom
listed above. She was in tears, wondering how she could continue living her life this way while being a mother of three children.
She had seen eight specialists who conducted every possible test.
Without a definite diagnosis, she was put on a variety of medications. Still miserable and as a last resort, she had scheduled an
appointment with the Mayo Clinic. She also had set up an appointment with me to see if I could help her.

Immediately, I suspected that since none of her tests proved
positive for any recognized condition in Western medicine and
since all of her symptoms were common with electromagnetic hypersensitivity (see Chapter 7), she was possibly being affected by
electromagnetic pollution. I lent her a Gauss meter (a hand-held
measuring device) to check for harmful electromagnetic frequencies (EMFs) throughout her house. She found the biggest problems
in her bedroom. A clock radio and cell phone plugged in on the
nightstand next to her head and the exercise machine and laptop
computer in the corner of the room all emitted high EMF frequencies. In addition, she realized a cell phone tower was located near
her house. All those frequencies were impacting her life and her
young family. Once she turned off all the electrical "traffic" in her
bedroom, her severe symptoms gradually disappeared.

This is such a common story. I spoke two years in a row at a career day at my kids' elementary school and was alarmed to discover
that when asked how many of the students had sleep problems,
more than half the students raised their hands. My next question
was, "How many of you are experiencing headaches and fatigue?"
Even more hands went up. Before I asked that question, I had suspected a fair percentage of the children might have experienced
such symptoms, but I was surprised at exactly *how* high the percentage was. Parents, listen on!

Earth Frequencies Versus Artificial, Man-Made Frequencies

Early in my business travels, I decided to accumulate frequent flier
miles so that I could visit new countries. It's important to know

that not only do you become a frequent flier, you also become a *frequency* flier. What exactly does that mean? It means that whichever man-made cage you choose—be it bus, plane, train, boat or car—you are *constantly* impacted by the frequency of energy around you.

When it comes to travel, you are exposed to man-made frequencies that run between 60 hertz and 2.45 gigahertz. Electromagnetic frequencies (EMFs) in this range challenge the very core of health in your body.

Every cell in your body, including your heart and brain cells, is designed for low-energy frequencies in the range of 5-25 hertz. These are the earth's normal frequencies. These frequencies are found most potently outdoors and especially near the ocean. The earth frequencies are the life-promoting sparks, along with air, water and minerals, which give all of life the charge to create energy, health and the good vibrations in your cells.

Every organ system in your body, especially your immune, endocrine and respiratory systems, requires these frequencies to function properly, optimally and to ensure sustainable health.

Nobel Prize-winner and German physicist Dr. Werner Heisenberg said it best when he described the earth's electromagnetic energy of the earth as the elemental energy on which all of life depends. It's important to note here that this life-supporting field has diminished greatly in terms of intensity in the past 60-plus years and is a major factor in the extinction of many species.

What frequencies are you around that are disharmonious? Your cell phone is at least 900 megahertz and your laptop is even higher. How about the frequencies emitted by your Wi-Fi, hair dryers, kitchen appliances or halogen lights? Be aware that most electromagnetic pollution cannot be seen, heard, felt, or tasted. However, when detected with special measuring devices such as Gauss meters, these frequencies create a high-intensity piercing sound, which is very uncomfortable to hear. Buy a Gauss meter and find out for yourself. (See Chapter 10.)

Imagine how you would feel staying in a dorm room in China, where outside your door you hear jackhammers, drills and hammers 24/7 for one full month. I have experienced this myself and hardly slept a wink. I felt anxious in a way that I had never known before. This is my best-ever example of dissonance during travel.

Thankfully, I spent most of my days in China working in the hospitals and traveling on the *only* day off, Sunday.

Take a moment and look at Figure 1A. This clearly represents the negative impact of harmful frequencies by which we are surrounded. Notice the red jiggly line around the earth. This is the benevolent magnetic field that surrounds the earth and shields you from solar flares, electrical storms and toxic particles.

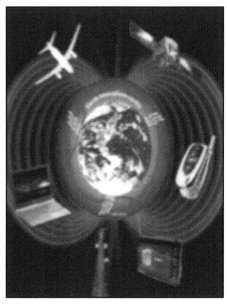

Figure 1A

In a very short time, we have transitioned from plow and farm to commercial markets and an industrialized, technological world where many of you as well as your loved ones are spending a majority of life indoors. You not only drive to work, but most of you work indoors 40-plus hours a week. The average American is now estimated to spend 90% of his or her lifetime indoors. If you find this hard to believe, track your outdoor time for seven straight days. You might be shocked by the results, as many of my patients have been. A client of mine recently reported, "I am blown away to discover that in seven days I was only outdoors for three solid hours. Ouch! This is not the way I want to live anymore."

For the next seven days, I encourage you to monitor how much time you are actually outdoors in the fresh air—if it is even available where you live! I know a very outdoorsy woman who often boasted of her outdoor life and, on my suggestion, she tracked one week of her life. After four hours of running that week, she calculated two additional hours spent outdoors, which totaled a slim six hours of outside time in a seven-day period. She cried out in disbelief when she did this exercise. Now it's your turn. For the next seven days, count the total hours you are outside.

So, if your body is designed for the earth's magnetic frequencies and instead you are living indoors for most of the time, where the average frequency is between 60 Hz and 1000 Hz, with air conditioning, electricity, Wi-Fi and radio frequencies reaching 2.45 GHz to 300 GHz (or *billions* of times per second), it is not surprising that travel and your "indoor lifestyle" can exhaust you and degrade your health in multiple ways. As Clinton Ober states in his book *Earthing*, we are all immersed in an unseen sea of human-generated electromagnetic fields. And in the documentary film *Full Signal*, Palestinian filmmaker Talal Jabari calls this EMF world the "biggest biological experiment ever" and the "hidden health epidemic" spreading among us.

Some well-known and respected authorities, including physicians Mehmet Oz, Joseph Mercola and Dietrich Klinghardt, have referred to these wireless technologies as the smoking gun of the 21st century. In other words, these unhealthy frequencies are contributing massively to the 30,000 diseases found in our world today.

Just 60 years ago, we saw advertisements promoting smoking with endorsements from medical doctors. Some of you might recall this statement from an advertisement: "More doctors smoke Camels than any other cigarette." Can you imagine commercials today saying that doctors prefer to experience cell phone and smart meter radiation more than any other type of radiation, just to increase the sale of phones and meters? Ridiculous.

Health writer Ann Louise Gittleman devoted an entire book called *Zapped* to this epidemic. We might not see, feel, taste, or smell these harmful frequencies, yet they are all around us and there is no escape! Just know that there are serious threats to our well-being from our electrosmog-ridden world.

Many of my patients have developed severe sensitivities to these artificial fields, and there is now a World Health Organization health category called "Electro-hypersensitivity." I have devoted Chapter 7 to this ever-growing epidemic among children, adults and our aging nation.

Dr. Magda Havas, also an expert in this field, is among the many scientists who have done extensive research proving that these artificial frequencies disrupt all aspects of your health. When I heard her speak at a lecture, she described the long list of symptoms caused by these frequencies, including the most common— fatigue, sleep issues, blood sugar imbalance, dizziness, gastrointestinal

distress, depression, memory problems, headaches and poor metabolism leading to obesity." She even claimed that EMFs have led
to a new "Type III Diabetes." We need our spark of healthy earth
EMFs, and we just aren't getting enough of it in our increasingly
toxic world.

Dr. Mark Hyman says it best: "Eighty thousand toxic chemicals have been released into our environment since the dawn of
the industrial revolution, and very few have been tested for their
long-term impact on human health. And let me tell you, the results
aren't pretty for those that have been tested." (1) Other than our
Electrosmog toxicity, pollution from geo-engineering, Bisphenol A
(BPA) in plastics, pesticides, mercury, lead and other heavy metal
toxins, countless xenobiotics also impact us. According to Wikipedia,
a xenobiotic is a chemical which is found in an organism but which
is not normally produced or expected to be present in it.

I hope you're starting to easily see how absolutely critical it is
for you to commit to a life of optimal health choices and not just
while traveling!

Are you ready to become a healthy frequency flier?

Remember how you felt after a long car ride. How often do you get
off the plane at your destination, glance at yourself in a mirror and
see how pale-faced, exhausted and foggy-headed you are, not to
mention that the gorgeous hairdo you spent time on that morning
is now in ruins? Or think about how you feel even after just one full
day inside a hotel at a business conference.

To give you an example of positive vibrations, think of how you
would feel listening to your favorite Beethoven or Mozart composi-
tions, or remember a time in your past when you felt totally in harmony and balanced after a three-hour hike in nature or just a few
hours on the beach. It is no wonder that sound frequencies have
become increasingly popular as a way of healing, with tuning forks,
live music performances and different types of sound therapy. These
modalities can create healthy frequencies in and around the body.

Remember these times and think of the ways that you can create and allow more of these kind of moments, especially while

traveling. This type of energy equals health. To repeat, our biological structure is designed just like nature, and just as with all living things on earth, we thrive when exposed to the very low frequencies of nature in the range of 0 to 30Hz.

I recommend to all my patients who travel that they seek healthy vibrations as often as possible while on their trip. What does this look like? Here are some ideas for you:

EIGHT STEPS TO HEALTHY, FREQUENT AND FREQUENCY TRAVEL

1. Refresh yourself by being outdoors as much as possible.

During breaks at meetings or even while hiking, find green grass and take your shoes and socks off so that you are able to literally ground yourself to the earth through the bottom of your feet. There is a powerful acupuncture point on the sole of your foot called "Gushing Spring" that is strongly rooting and, when activated, helps you return to your connection with the earth. Some alternate names for this point are "Earth Surge" and "Earth Thoroughfare." Simply walking barefoot or putting your bare feet on a rock is a quick way to neutralize stress in your body and mind.

A good way to view this is to imagine your unhealthy cells resembling shriveled raisins, which turn into voluptuous grapes as they are nourished by "gushing springs" of pure energy. This is what happens when you give your cells what they need. Dr. Linus Pauling, two-time Nobel Prize winner in physics, says: "When your cells are

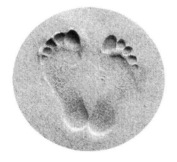

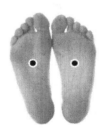

The Goal of Earthing is to duplicate the bioelectrical effect of walking barefoot on wet sand

Kidney 1 acupuncture point

"Gushing Spring" name of point on bottom of feet

healthy, you feel good, your immune system is stronger and you have energy." I suggest to every single flight attendant, pilot and patient, as well as you, HCT, to get outside for at least 20 minutes when you get to your destination to dust off from the onslaught of harmful frequencies and radiation in order to ground your body. Yes, even before you sleep.

2. **Refuel your cells with nature by getting into healthy bodies of water, when available.**

Plan your trips around your favorite beach, hot mineral springs or a lake or river destination. Your body loves clean water, and many hot springs offer a multitude of healing properties, from pain relief to stress relief. I have asked the question, "Where do you feel the best?" to thousands of people, whether on my treatment tables or while publicly speaking. Hands down, a day at the beach gets the highest vote. I bet you know exactly why. See the "Ultimate Health Formula" below.

3. **Embody The 8 Pathways known as the Ultimate Health Formula (UHF).**

The Ultimate Health Formula, as outlined in this book, is the sum total of smart and conscious travel. In other words: your personal power + earth frequencies + lots of healthy water + optimal nutrition + movement + presence in the moment (including your best positive thoughts) + awareness of your interconnectedness to people, place and the universe = **Ultimate Health**.

4. **Bring your favorite essential oils and take a warm bath on arrival.**

Choose 100% natural essential oils to recalibrate your energy, reboot your immune system and help you with digestive issues after a long journey. My favorite blend for travel is Thieves® essential oil blend by Young Living, which is great for infection and clearing congested air. The mixture contains clove, cinnamon, eucalyptus and rosemary. I also carry lemon, peppermint, lavender and clove oils when I travel. (For more information, see Chapter 9.)

Like many of you, I can't wait for the day when perfumes are banned from air travel. Imagine getting reminders to "think of your neighbor and please refrain from wearing perfume or cologne during today's flight." This might cause quite a stir, but it certainly would take one thing off the long list of toxins we breathe in during travel.

This suggestion might make some of you cringe, but most commercial perfumes and lotions you put on your body are synthetic toxins that are setting you up for serious health issues. Remember, your skin is your largest organ and *everything* you put on it is quickly absorbed into your body. To be safe, if you cannot *eat* it, do not put it on your body. Organic virgin coconut oil or pure olive oil on your skin is an excellent choice. Remember to be kind to your liver, your detoxifying powerhouse, by choosing natural products instead of man-made toxins.

5. Chant, pray, listen to music and breathe deeply.

This brings about the best vibrations and frequencies for your mind and body. Think of the song "Good Vibrations" from the Beach Boys. Doesn't that song just put you in the best mood? Your favorite choice of music can be your best antidote against the worst turbulence, a bad mood after a flight delay or a sore back after two hours of car travel. My dear friend Celeste Yacoboni, author of the book *How Do You Pray?*, has this to offer: "Your every breath can be a prayer of forgiveness for the loud mouth on the bus or the person in a hurry who cut in front of you in line or the waitperson that didn't give you the attention that you deserved. Every breath is a prayer, a prayer of gratitude for your amazing life. As you breathe in the support of the earth and energy of the heavens, know you are home wherever you are."

6. Drink the best possible water.

Just add a pinch of sea salt to help rehydrate your body before, during and after travel. Water can immediately give you a boost. The challenge is that most of us do not absorb the water we drink because it lacks the natural earth frequencies and proper minerals necessary for us to absorb the water into our cells. This is the purpose of the sea salt, which is rich in minerals and trace minerals. (See Chapter 4 for additional information.)

7. Invest in reputable products that help neutralize harmful frequencies.

This would include Earthing sheets, EMF protective pendants or crystals, shields and protective clothes. Invest in the best pulsed electromagnetic frequency (PEMF) wellness devices, which mimic the earth's frequencies and quickly recharge your body's "cell batteries." (See Chapter 10 for more information and suggestions.)

8. Invest in your stress resiliency.

As an HCT, you want a clear game plan for how to handle stressful delays, cancellations, getting through security or finding yourself stuck in traffic on a freeway in L.A. Seriously, write a note to yourself from your higher-evolved self about the three things you commit to do on a regular basis when the you-know-what hits the fan while traveling (Pathway 8).

For me, when travel takes an unexpected turn, I always ask myself what is the worst thing that can happen? Just that inquiry alone lowers my stress immediately. Even my two teenagers have adopted this strategy. Secondly, I become aware of my breath to bring my thoughts into coherence with the present moment. Thirdly, I feel my feet planted on the earth wherever I am and I ground myself. As soon as I accept what is, I can let go and move forward.

I frequently prescribe De-Stress, an all-natural product that is a precursor to Gaba (an important amino acid that supports healthy moods and relieves anxiety) for the highly stressed traveler and for people who have a fear of flying. (See Chapter 9.)

Also, why not keep a laminated, written copy of your goals and life-purpose handy in the glove compartment of your car or packed in your carry-on luggage? Always remember what you are living for, realizing that life and the timing of things are rarely perfect and that, in the end, the stress you put yourself through will barely be remembered even days later. Chill, marvel in the WOW of the unknown and challenge yourself to be your best, most *resilient* person under the worst of circumstances. In a book called *The Turning Point*, author Gregg Braden calls this "expanded resilience," referring to strategies of resilient thinking about our finances, unexpected events and personal and spiritual transformations that expand us into even more conscious and aware human beings.

Love and Nourish Your Electric Body

Understanding the electrical nature of your body may be the most important thing you need to know, not only to restore your health but also to allow you to make choices that support the electrical nature of your entire system. Read on and get excited to really grasp this so you can literally turn your health around and sustain the vitality you desire.

Did you know that 70 to 85% of your body is made of water and minerals (sodium, potassium, magnesium, among others)? Please take note: Your body is more bio-identical to the earth than anything else. *So it makes complete sense that what is good for your body is good for the earth, and what is good for the earth is good for your body.* This combination of water + minerals and, yes, positive thoughts and real foods (which creates an alkaline environment) is what makes your body a natural conductor of electricity. Your body's electrical system controls the function of every cell. On the other hand, negative thinking, dehydration and processed foods create a very acidic environment in your body that makes you a poor conductor of electricity, and therefore your health becomes compromised.

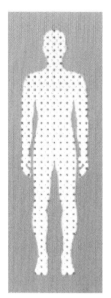

Figure 1D

First and foremost, we need our system to be supported by the earth's magnetic field. This is what I call the "holy spark" that ensures that our biology and body chemistry are functioning optimally. Now you can understand why you need to walk barefoot as much as possible.

This may also help you understand why artificial electrical sources are so toxic to your health. To be well and healthy, it is essential for every tissue in your body to have highly functioning cells and especially cell membranes. As Louis Pasteur once put it, we are only as healthy as our 70 trillion cells.

A high-functioning cell should be perfectly round and free from neighboring cells. Clumped cells, on the other hand, indicate inflammation and oxygen deprivation, as evidenced in dark field microscopy. For healthy function, the cell wall should be thick, intact and free from heavy metals and unhealthy parasites, yeast, bacteria and fungus. (See Figure 1F.)

Sustain health in your body by creating healthy cells 24/7

To clearly understand the electrical nature of your body, think of your cells as individual batteries. In fact, your body is one big battery. If your battery is dim and low functioning, you will feel miserable. When your battery is charged on a regular basis you feel vibrant and alive. In order to have healthy, charged cells, you need the electromagnetic field of the earth combined with air, water and minerals, primarily from your diet. Your energy will remain vibrant when you are getting enough of these four essential ingredients. When you are deficient in any one of these, it's likely that your health will deteriorate.

Bruce Lipton, a world-renowned leader in cellular biology and quantum physics research and bestselling author of *The Biology of Belief*, has proven that it is primarily our internal environment, not our DNA, that shapes the development of our cells. In other words, your food choices as well as your thoughts and intentions have more impact on your state of health than your genetics (Pathways 3, 6 and 7).

A healthy cell membrane is one of the most important indicators of your overall health. In the book *Healing Is Voltage*, Dr. Jerry Tennant measures a healthy cell membrane in terms of millivolts (mv). The higher the voltage of your cell membrane, the better health you have. The values he attributes to healthy versus unhealthy cells are as follows, based on ideal blood pH of 7.35-7.4. This is a synonym of -20 to -25 millivolts.

Healthy cells: -50 mv (optimal range to make new cells)

Normal cells: -25 mv

Cancer cells: +30 mv (cancer and disease occurs)

His personal journey from near death to completely turning his life around is remarkable: turning his cellular voltage "on" saved his life. Now he tours the globe speaking and teaching and has invented his own tool, called the Biomodulator, to help increase health to each of your cells. In Chapter 10, I will discuss technologies like the Tennant Biomodulator, which is a precision medical instrument used for symptomatic relief and management of chronic, intractable pain. It does this by charging your cells' voltage potential and renewing under-functioning cells. To hear my recent interview with Dr. Tennant, visit www.healthytravelerssummit.com.

Envision your cells once again looking like voluptuous juicy grapes (-50 to -70 mv) compared to a clump of sticky raisins. You have to be 100% committed to producing vibrant grape cells on a daily basis, so you can avoid being like most Americans who are feeling wired, tired and sick. Perhaps it is safe to say that we have become a "wired, tired, stressed and depressed" world, but that certainly doesn't have to be the case moving forward.

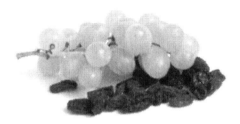

Figure 1E

Figure 1E illustrates the analogy of high voltage cells (grapes) that absorb oxygen, water and nutrients well, on top of clumped cells (raisins) with low cell membrane voltage that lack proper oxygen utilization. These clumped cells are how your cells may look after a long flight or car ride without proper hydration and nutritious foods as quality fuel.

Activate health rather than disease with healthy food choices during travel and before you leave your house. What one change will you make today that will increase the voltage or energetic frequency of your cells?

Frequency matters

"Everything is energy" is one of Einstein's most famous quotes. You might have heard that energy medicine is the medicine of the future. What does this mean? It means that there is an energetic field in and around you and all living things, and the medicine of the future aims to correct this field *first*. You may be unable to see the energetic field, yet scientists have proven that it exists. This is your "electric" body. Again, turning on this field with the best possible frequencies like music, laughter, dance and the eight suggestions listed previously will often return you to health and happiness.

With modern, sophisticated technology such as Kirlian photography, thermography, live blood cell analysis and even pulse oximeter readings, it is possible to detect immediate energy shifts in the body after acupuncture, chiropractic work, chanting and other energetic modalities. The brighter picture of the two shown below, taken after lying on a Magnetic Resonance Stimulation mat (MRS), an energetic healing modality, indicates a considerable increase in energy flow, vitality and overall distribution of *qi* (life force). Read more about this in Chapter 10.

The first photo reveals the state of a person's tired battery cells before exposure to a healthy earthing field. The second photo illustrates what happens after the healthy energy field of the MRS mat has been applied for just eight minutes. Hydration, good thoughts and healthy foods also increase the healthy voltage of your cells.

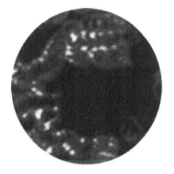

Before MRS   After MRS

Figure 1F

When I insert an acupuncture needle into a point on your body, it changes the frequency and the electrical nature of your body immediately. One needle can often relieve pain simply by changing the energy flow in a particular area on your body. Acupuncture points are part of an "electronic grid" in our bodies. Health is achieved when the grid is functioning properly. If there is a so-called "power outage" on the grid, we develop health issues.

In addition to acupuncture, there are many Complementary Alternative Medicine modalities (CAM), such as massage, herbs, biofeedback, acupressure, Tapping and numerous other therapies that restore the balance of your sensitive electrical system, as seen in Figure 1F. We will cover this in more depth in Chapter 10. These treatments can be very helpful when you are experiencing health issues. Of course it's obvious, but I do need to say that you should see your doctor or go to the nearest emergency room for any serious issues.

What about radiation?

This is a major topic, so I want you to have a rudimentary under-standing of what radiation is and how it impacts you in terms of travel and daily life. There are two types of radiation. One is non-ionizing, low-energy radiation that is considered less harmful. This kind of radiation includes wave-charged particles, which come from sun exposure and other cosmic sources and is also found in the soil and in the air. The more harmful type of radiation that causes cel-lular breakdown is high-energy ionizing radiation, and it's found in CT scans, X-rays, airport security scanning, certain cosmic radia-tion during flights, microwave ovens and wireless technologies, to name only a few.

I've already told you that you are exposed to the equivalent of one hospital X-ray procedure while on a flight across the U.S. The exact biological consequences of ionizing radiation are highly de-batable. However, there are ways to measure harmful radiation, and it has been determined that the amount of cosmic radiation you are exposed to while flying depends on your altitude and how far away you are from the equator.

Those of us who live at higher altitudes (like Santa Fe, New Mexico, Denver, Colorado, or Mount Shasta, California) are exposed to higher levels of radiation on a daily basis. One of the best ways to avoid high levels of radiation while flying is to sit further away from the window during the day or if you do have a window seat, close the window cover. As often as possible, take evening flights after sundown when the radiation levels are the lowest.

By following The 8 Pathways, you will keep your body in op-timal health. Make sure to consume a high-water, plant-based or-ganic diet, rich in antioxidants, to best protect your body from these types of radiation. This includes foods rich in iodine, such as algae, marine minerals and seaweed. Astaxanthin is an antioxidant de-rived from algae that is 65 times more powerful than Vitamin C at scavenging free radicals in your body. Vitamin D3 and Glutathione in the form of N-Acetyl Cysteine (NAC) or a liposomal delivery sys-tem (see Chapter 9) will help to protect you from regular radiation exposure.

At the beginning of this chapter, I shared an unpleasant ex-ample of disharmony while traveling in China. But I consider my time in the Masai Mara in Kenya, the great temples and pyramids in Egypt and the Sacred Valley of Peru to be my most harmonious travel experiences in terms of good vibrations and frequencies.

My trip to Kenya included my first-ever safari experience. The highlight, for sure, was seeing prides of lions and elephant families mingling around the acacia trees. We would stop, look and listen to the sounds of lions in the distance and hear the loud call of the elephants. One day, a crocodile moving through the brush beside the water caught my eye. I felt this shift in my body, and I became part of the natural world around me. I was very aware of the birds, the insects, the acacia trees and all the animals following their own innate rhythm: moving, eating, hunting and communicating in their own unique way. I felt privileged to be there and to observe their way of living in harmony. These amazing travel moments remind me as an HCT to never forget the simplicity of life and to recharge by reconnecting to nature's frequencies as often as possible (Pathway 2).

So why not be healthy and stay well to take advantage of all the world of travel offers? It is all about being conscious, aware and active on your journey. After all, we are all *traveling* through this life each and every day, so cheers to creating the best *life* experience you can have: one that is fulfilling, inspired and full of life-promoting frequencies as a *frequent* flier.

Call to action:

- Before and during each and every trip, take the time to plan ways to minimize unhealthy frequencies in order to sustain your energetic health. For example, don't put laptop computers on your lap. Put them on a table instead. Text or use your speaker phone instead of putting your phone near your head. If possible, turn off Wi-Fi every night before you go to bed, because its radiation extends 600 feet, and you don't want that to include your bed.

- Journal about where in the world you like to travel. Next write down memorable places you have been to, where you feel the absolute best. Notice your surroundings. How do you feel in this environment when you wake up and go to bed at night?

- Be aware of times when you feel full of energy and truly alive. How have your nourished yourself with foods, thoughts, water and movement?

- If you think you can't truly be away from technology, test yourself by booking a river trip or traveling to a remote area where you can completely disconnect. Consider doing this a few times a year to fully charge your body, mind and spirit

Chapter 2

Thrive as You Travel with Optimal Nutrition

Let food be thy medicine and medicine be thy food.
~ Hippocrates

The major problems in the world are the result of the difference
between the way nature works and the way people think.
~ Gregory Bateson

What do you think determines your overall health more than any other factor? Take a moment to think about this question. Did you know that at least 80% of your overall health status is diet and food related? You don't have to look too far beyond what you're eating to solve most of your health issues.

Have you noticed there is a revolution going on when it comes to educating the general population on the hazards of eating the Standard American Diet (SAD)? I believe that poor diet, one that is depleted in essential vitamins, minerals, amino acids and other nutrients, is the root of this disease epidemic. New films, books and online programs regularly address this important issue, often provocatively, including Katie Couric's *Fed Up*, Morgan Spurlock's *Supersize Me*, Jeffrey Hays' *Bought*, Robert Kenner's, *Food Inc.*, Eric

Schlosser's *Fast Food Nation*, Jeffrey Smith's *Genetic Roulette*, Pedram Shojai's two films *Vitality* and *Origins* and Dave Asprey's newly released *Moldy*. These and other films and books are examples of conscious media aimed at educating us about the dangers of America's food and living in an increasingly toxic world.

When it comes to being your best health care advocate (Pathway 1), your number one priority is to eat real food (Pathway 2).

In terms of diet, you may feel more confused than ever with new programs coming out daily on newsstands, on the Internet, in bookstores and from your personal fitness trainer. I am often asked, "Should I go with the South Beach Diet or maybe the Clean or the Paleo Diet?"

You can do yoga and meditate daily, but without a healthy diet, you are not feeding your brain, heart and every cell in your body and providing what is essential for your optimal and sustained performance. Granted, meditation, yoga and movement are good medicine, yet even these are best when paired with a clean diet.

Based on working with thousands of patients and devouring all the latest research, I can say without any doubt and more than any other factor, that your overall health is determined not only by what you eat, but also by what you digest and absorb. Instead of saying, "You are what you eat," it would be more accurate to say, "You are what you digest." You might be eating healthy foods, but if the food you're eating is not properly digested and assimilated, you are missing the proper nourishment you need.

As we age, we often experience a general decline in our ability to digest foods due to a deficiency of a broad range of digestive enzymes, including hydrochloric acid, protease, lipase, cellulase, amylase and pancreatin, that are necessary for you to process vital nutrients. Be sure to travel with digestive enzymes and avoid bloating, gas and other upsets after eating. In Chinese medicine, a healthy gut is absolutely necessary for a healthy body and spirit, so don't throw junk thoughts and food into your body. (See Chapter 9.)

I am often asked in my practice, "What food should I eat, Robyn, especially since I travel so often?" Or, "What diet or nutrition plan should I consider when there are so many to choose from?" The world of nutrition and dieting is a multi-billion dollar industry that is often more interested in profits than in fostering your optimal health. As an HCT, you know this and can choose to free yourself from the temptation to support this aspect of the food industry, even when traveling!

In Oriental Medicine, we view food as medicine. You have a unique genetic makeup. By viewing your tongue, feeling your pulses and taking a thorough medical history, it is often clear what foods are best for you and your overall constitution. One size does not fit all. Some patients do well with hot and spicy foods, while others need more cooling foods. What I see more than anything are tongues that are covered with a white-yellowish coating, which is often indicative of yeast/fungal overgrowth in the body. Overconsumption of sugar and processed food is the root cause and sets you up for all types of health issues, from diabetes to joint pain and digestive discomfort.

Michael Pollan, author of *The Omnivore's Dilemma*, sums up all nutritional research in these simple principles: "Eat food. Not too much. Mostly plants. In fact, you need to know nothing else to be vibrantly healthy."

Keep it simple by getting back to the basics of nature and how your body operates best.

After reading Chapter 1 and understanding healthy frequencies and your "electrical body," you already know that you will thrive when your cells are high functioning and have a healthy voltage. Your body and every cell inside you require high-energy food that is alive. There is truth to the adage, "An apple a day keeps the doctor away." Something as simple as a non-GMO apple or orange right off the tree holds the energy that your body needs.

Your body thrives with fresh organic greens from your home garden and local farms. As you eat high-voltage food, it creates a symphony of happy cells in your body, rather than sticky, inflamed cells that are a result of fake, dead and processed food. In other words, your "electrical body" is always looking for foods and nutrition that keep your cell batteries charged, thus promoting high and sustained energy. If you care to find out about your best nutritional blueprint, contact a holistic practitioner or an Integrative M.D. who can do an overall evaluation, including lab work and a food allergy/sensitivity test so you will feel confident knowing what best food feeds and fuels your unique body. The food choices you make, daily, determine your overall health, vitality and longevity and are your best *insurance*, or protection from any possible disease.

Food and International Travel

Are you like many who love to travel to experience savory and exotic foods from around the world? Then the last thing you want is to be on a limited diet. Perhaps you have fond memories of eating cheese and butter-drenched crêpes in Paris, or the best homemade pasta you've ever tasted in Rome. How about the time you found yourself in a tucked-away bakery on a side alley in Malta? I'll bet you can remember salivating as you eyed the best pastries you had ever seen. Or you might have been sitting in a café, eating moussaka as you overlooked the Mediterranean Sea in Greece. These are moments you will never forget. They not only feed your body but your mind and spirit as well.

As you prepare for present and future travel, practice self-care, knowing that every morsel you put in your mouth contributes to how well you feel. Very often, a plane, train, bus, motorcycle or any type of travel plan becomes your ticket to a feast of unhealthy food. It starts with rushing out the door without breakfast and with little option other than choosing fast food, convenient sugar-filled foods and beverages. Many vacations start and end on a sugar high. It is common to come home from a nine-day trip in Europe or a weekend sports trip with the best of memories but also a few extra pounds and an uncomfortable bloat around your tummy. Can you remember a vacation or two like that? "I am still holding onto an extra 25 pounds of weight from my trip to Italy six months ago," a patient recently lamented. As you follow Pathway 1 in this book and become the CEO of your overall health, you will *retrain* yourself to have a different mindset about travel and your dietary choices.

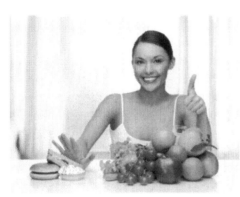

In Europe, the food is healthier than it is in the U.S. For example, you can find excellent dairy sources in European countries that you cannot find in America because, unlike in the U.S., European grocery stores and restaurants carry unpasteurized, grass-fed dairy products. I personally refrain from dairy because it does not make my gut feel very good, yet I did not have the same problem when I traveled to Ireland, Spain and France. Do your homework and learn about the sources of the dairy products you eat.

When it comes to genetically modified organisms (GMOs), you have much less detective work to do as most GMO foods are banned from the European Union (EU) The U.S. should do the same in my opinion, as GMO foods are extremely destructive to our gut health and our brain for that matter, so it is best to avoid them anywhere, as a general rule, if you truly care about your health. (See the Call to Action at the end of this chapter for more information about GMO foods.)

Consider ways you can enjoy enormous eating pleasure while traveling and still take care of yourself at the same time. Imagine feeling energized, engaged and alert when you make better food choices. In the end, this will contribute to your extraordinary travel experience as well as a sustained and strong immune system.

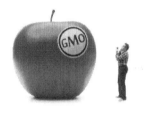

Food is one of the most enjoyable ways to experience the cultures of the world, and for many, travel in this way melts any sense of separation you might feel from your extended family. We are all connected and this, too, is a valuable aspect of being a Healthy Conscious Traveler, feeding your soul as you cultivate rich relationships on a global level.

The uncertainty food factor with travel

The next time you open your refrigerator or look in your cabinets at home, check if you are seeing your best possible *food pharmacy*, one that feeds your whole body. Do the choices you have made support your decision to be the CEO of your optimal health care? Do these foods in front of you give you energy or do you see too many canned and packaged foods that provide very little nutritional value?

What percentage of the food in your house is life promoting, alive and full of the natural vitamins and minerals from the earth?

These are the same questions that you want to ask yourself when you face hundreds of food choices in airports, bus and train stations or convenience stores along the road.

If you are accustomed to a well-stocked, healthy kitchen, the uncertainty of travel and not having your comfort foods within reach can be daunting. It becomes easier to make wise choices when you consider the voltage factor. A cheeseburger and French fries from McDonald's has far less voltage than a banana or a small salad. Of course, it would be better if the food you eat is organic, which unfortunately, is not common in American fast-food stores and most restaurants, for that matter, due to the fact that organic food prices are somewhat higher.

I am happy to report that the movement for healthier food choices in the travel industry is accelerating in some areas more than others. I was amazed to recently come across a gourmet health food store in the Salt Lake City airport. It was a feast for my eyes and health-conscious palate to see freshly made organic salads and lots of gluten-free options as well. I had the best-tasting tabouli salad of my life from that store. A few gates farther on, for the first time ever in an airport, I came across my favorite Gingerberry Synergy drink. For any of you fellow kombucha lovers, you can only

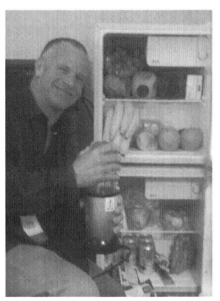

imagine how exciting this was. The bubbly, sweet taste was the perfect antidote to a four-day business trip. If you are new to this beverage, let me enlighten you. The label reads "living food for the living body with a unique blend of proprietary probiotics and powerful antioxidants designed to nourish your body from the inside out." Now that's what I'm talkin' about!

My HCT friend Gregg Schulman's refrigerator is stocked with healthy food at the Marriott hotel during a recent conference.

Like Gregg, you can become part of this Self-care Revolution movement for travelers today!

In 2013 my business, Santa Fe Soul Center for Optimal Health, launched the Self-care Revolution, which aims to transform lives and health care, one person at a time. Health and wealth advocate Steve Rose, had this to say: "The Self-care Revolution is on the cutting edge of people taking responsibility for their health, wealth and state of happiness." Joining in your personal self-care revolution is certainly a theme of this book. To get access to this free online course, which features more than 150 experts in the health, wellness and fitness world, visit www.jointheselfcare revolution.com. To learn specifically about healthy travel, visit the popular www.healthytravelerssummit.com.

The Cost of Getting Sick Today

Why are you, as the HCT, committed to The 8 Pathways in this time of unprecedented change? The best answer is that it costs too much for you to get sick, not only in terms of your dollars but your energy, your relationships and more. Did you know a study done at George Washington University found that the annual cost of being obese for women is $4,787 and for men $2,626?(1) According to *The New York Times*, if you were diagnosed with diabetes today, you could expect to pay an additional $6,000 per year in medical expenses, and for an Alzheimer's diagnosis, at least $30,000 per year. (2) According to recent estimates, the average person diagnosed with cancer will spend $300,000 in health care expenses. I have known countless people who have spent far more than this for cancer treatments. This is another reason why preventative health care is at the *top* of the HCT list of daily values. Your health is truly your wealth!

The cost of a common, undiagnosed disease

Could this be your undiagnosed health issue? A woman came into my office, stressed and in pain. She was running out of money after spending $15,000 on health care trying to solve her severe abdominal pain. It was clear, after an initial exam, that she had inflammation in her gut. I treated her with acupuncture and herbs. To help her solve her problem, I also encouraged her to take a specific blood test. My hunch was correct; when the results came in, it was definite that she had celiac disease. This meant that she was severely allergic to gluten, which is found in many breads, sauces and packaged foods.

She is among many who suffer severely with this condition. Dr. Tom O'Bryan, known as the "gluten doctor," shared in one of our interviews for the Self-care Revolution that 2% of the population has celiac disease and about 70% is sensitive to gluten. In both cases, people who ingest gluten suffer miserably with all types of gut pain, gas, headaches, fertility issues and much more. Celiac disease and gluten sensitivity are perfect examples of how food can be the root cause of disease. "Undiagnosed celiac disease continues to be a silent killer among many people as they live miserable lives, often taking prescription drugs for the symptoms and not the cause." Dr. O'Bryan says.

I feel obligated to test all people who come in with digestive complaints by using a celiac panel and a food allergy/sensitivity test. I believe that it's essential to educate my patients about their unique nutritional needs and the role food intolerance plays in health maintenance. This is one of the best ways to put an end to a lot of unnecessary pain and suffering that people often endure throughout their lives.

Imagine restoring a future of good moods, happy tummies, sharp minds and eradicating major inflammation by simply discovering whether you have celiac disease or food allergies. If you have any of the symptoms of celiac disease, such as abdominal pain, rashes, brain fog, bloating, weight gain, or recurring sinus infections, please get tested as soon as possible. May you become one of many who defeat their illness and regain their life by eliminating gluten and following a primarily plant- and earth-based diet. See Chapter 10 for details.

As an HCT, three of the most important processes you may care to manage beautifully now and throughout your life, are inflammation, blood sugar levels and, yes, your stress level. It is a fact that you and your loved ones are living longer, but not necessarily better lives. It is now more common than ever to know someone who has a crippled body, yet a sharp mind. As an aging nation, we are seeing more and more people who are living well into their nineties, yet at the same time relying on multiple pharmaceutical drugs and plagued for years with pain, depression and uncontrollable blood sugar levels.

There is no better way to manage healthy inflammation, blood sugar levels and ultimately stress, than to "choose wisely with your fork," says Dr. Mark Hyman and to grab what Mother Earth provides for you such as fruits, vegetables, nuts, seeds and legumes. Dr. Hyman is one amazing doctor whose mission is to restore medicine to a true health-care system. I highly recommend all his books and information.

Dr. Hyman states, "What you put at the end of your fork is more powerful medicine than anything you will find at the bottom of a pill bottle. Food is the most powerful medicine available to heal chronic disease, which will account for over 50 million deaths and cost the global economy $47 trillion by 2030. All you need to do is eat your medicine and think of your grocery store as your pharmacy."(3) Great advice!

INFLAMMATION IN THE BODY AND INFLAMMATORY FOODS TO ELIMINATE

Did you know that you create inflammation in your body simply by living a stressful life? Travel can be a source of stress for many. Inflammation is a natural and necessary response in the body whenever we encounter harmful and consistent stress, germs or when we injure ourselves.

Inflammation also is a result of our processed and chemicalized diet. When this occurs, our immune system steps in to fight foreign invaders and attempts to bring our body back into balance so that we can heal. Inflammatory chemicals are produced during an immune response that can be harmful to our tissues, but antioxidants in our foods, such as vitamins A, C, D and E, can reduce this response and restore order to our tissues.

I like what actor George Burns had to say about it when he once quipped that he would live forever because he was full preservatives. HCT, it is always good to have a sense of humor!

Here are some tips for better nutrition:

Avoid white sugar! Did you know that the average American is now consuming *150 pounds of sugar* per year? Know that it is poisonous to the body and accelerates aging. A better choice might be 100% organic pure cane sugar (Non-GMO) or local honey or organic maple syrup used in strict moderation. Sugar is addictive and known to cause all kinds of diseases, from diabetes and obesity to memory loss, heart disease and more.

Refrain from all synthetic sugar substitutes, such as those usually found in diet sodas and thousands of other packaged foods. It is important to read all ingredient labels before consuming these processed foods. These unnatural chemical substitutes are harmful and have been proven to cause health problems, including memory loss, obesity and other nervous disorders. Nutrasweet (Aspartame), Splenda (Sucralose) and these chemicals with many other names contain "excitotoxins," and they *excite* or stimulate your neural cells to death and are rapidly metabolized into methanol and other potent neurotoxins.

The *sweetener alternative* stevia is your best choice for a healthy sugar substitute and is better than xylitol, sorbitol or mannitol, which are sugar alcohols and often cause gastric and intestinal upsets. Stevia is 200 times stronger than sugar, without all the side effects. There is also a new alternative sweetener on the market called "Just Like Sugar." It is all natural, made with chicory and orange peel and can be used in baking.

Agave has also been known to have high levels of high fructose corn syrup (HFCS) in it and is not recommended. Agave has to go through a heavy chemical process to become a syrup and thus has many of the same effects on your body as HFCS.

Avoid processed foods, fast foods and buffets that are full of hidden chemicals like food colors, preservatives and hidden artificial flavors found in biscuits, pastries, sauce-laden meats, French fries and other fried foods that are cooked in rancid oils.

Ice cream and most other pasteurized dairy products are hard on your digestive system and often produce mucous. Many people are allergic to the casein in dairy, which is the cause of many sinus and gut issues in all age groups. Raw dairy from a reputable source is a great alternative. Your best alternative is milk, ice cream and yogurt made from coconut milk. Try it, you might be amazed by how good it tastes!

Avoid almost all snack foods at rest stops while driving and in airports and airplanes while flying, especially low-fat and low-sugar types, because of the chemicals used in processing. Most are full of chemicals and hydrogenated oils that take over two months to fully break down in your body. Imagine that!

Avoid high-sodium canned soups. Canned foods and most processed foods are essentially dead food with additives, including preservatives, coloring, GMO ingredients and hydrogenated oils that can destroy your health, not to mention the fact that many cans are lined with Bisphenol A (BPA), a toxic hormone-disrupting chemical.

Many energy and sports bars are full of whey, soy, peanuts, dry milk, bad oils and fake sugars that make these equivalent to an unhealthy candy bar. Check all the ingredients before you purchase to make sure you are not sensitive or allergic to them. Avoid all food bars with any type of food dyes or hydrogenated oils. We recommend the Self-care Revolution bars (see Chapter 10).

Stay away from soy products and all genetically modified foods, such as soy, corn, canola oil, cottonseed, sugar beets, apples, potatoes, Hawaiian papaya and some zucchini and yellow squash. Most soy is genetically modified and it has been known to have phytates, which are very difficult to digest and can affect the thyroid, causing hypothyroidism. "There is no joy in soy," says J. J. Virgin, celebrity nutritionist and fitness trainer.

Avoid these oils: corn, canola, soy, sunflower, safflower and walnut oils. These oils have a higher polyunsaturated fat content and are prone to forming dangerous lipid peroxides when exposed to air and heat and cause inflammation in your body. Your best choice is to use only grass-fed butter (great source of vitamin K2, CLA and omega-3s), organic, extra-virgin coconut oil and organic, cold-pressed extra-virgin olive oil.

Avoid soda, caffeinated drinks and alcohol. These drinks also increase inflammation and cause imbalances in your blood sugar.

White bread and gluten products often contain anti-nutrients, such as lectins, that damage the gut, increase intestinal permeability and cause allergic conditions. Bromine is used to treat flour, and since bromine and iodine are almost identical from a molecular standpoint, bromine can occupy the receptor sites for iodine in the thyroid. This can cause all kinds of chaos in your gut, thyroid and adrenals.

Yes, stress causes inflammation too, so be kind to your adrenal glands. Your adrenal glands are part of your endocrine glandular system, and they are the size of a walnut and sit on top of each of your kidneys. These glands are small yet powerful, as they control fluid balance and blood sugar levels and produce hormones that keep your body functioning in a dynamic balance amid whatever external or internal changes or challenges you meet. How well you live depends, to a large degree, on how well your adrenal glands function. HCT, take care of your adrenals by managing your stress, your moods, your energy and by taking many of the supplements you will see listed in Chapter 8.

A clean diet, meditation, breathing exercises and proper rest are also essential for healthy adrenal glands.

Now let's pause for a moment to reflect on everything you've learned and to further integrate what's been shared here, so that you can become more pro-active as an HCT. Take a few minutes to read and answer the following questions:

1. **How would you rate your overall state of health today? Rate yourself from 1 to 10, with 1 being the worst and 10 being your best and most optimal health state.**

	Rating (1 – 10) 10 is best	Comments
Overall Energy		
Immune Health		
Digestive System		
Nervous System		
Mental State		

2. **Close your eyes for a few minutes and scan your body while asking yourself this question: "Where will I be and how will I feel in the next five years if I make better choices with food, exercise and my thoughts?" Take as much time as you need. Write down your reflections in the space provided here.**

_____

_____

_____

_____

3. Use your imagination to travel to twenty years from now and see yourself having your annual physical, including a blood test. What is the outcome you want to see on that date? As an HCT, you know that you have tremendous power to shape and direct your overall health *at all times*. What will you change about your diet and lifestyle *now*, to prevent any possible diagnosis, knowing that disease occurs as a result of the cumulative effect of your daily choices over several years?

_____

_____

_____

_____

Now that you've taken a moment to reflect on your present and future health, move forward with a sense of self-empowerment as you make positive health choices that bring you to "Pleasure Island." This is that place where you get to live each day as you enjoy the benefits of following The 8 Pathways of the Healthy and Smart Traveler.

The pain of not following these simple pathways, on the other hand, is immense. Did you know that, soon, one out of two people might be diagnosed with cancer in their lifetime, according to the American Cancer Society? Please let this sink in without fear, but with simple awareness and consciousness of what is possible, knowing you have the power to prevent this from happening. I am being *bold* here, as a *Self-care Revolutionary*, because it is time that you commit to preventative health care and live each day with passion and intelligence to carry out your most incredible living legacy possible.

It is time to express your unique blueprint, without hiding behind disbeliefs and fears or masking your brilliance with unconscious behaviors and addictions.

The 3 Ps: Proper Preparation Prevents Unnecessary Travel Stress, Illness and Fatigue

1. Plan for international travel and long days of car travel by buying enough food and healthy snacks to cover you for 24 to 48 hours that can easily fit in a soft lunch container with a small frozen gel pack. Otherwise, you are left with what airports, airlines, fast food restaurants and convenience stores offer you, which is not much!

See *The Healthy Conscious Traveler's Food Guide* for recipes and suggestions for the best foods to travel with.

2. Prepare ahead of time and start building your immune system two weeks before your departure with a high-quality probiotic and a nutrient-rich and high-water content diet. You can choose from the nine foods listed below: all low-inflammatory foods that are also low in sugar.

3. Pack bags of dry goods like nuts, dried fruit, organic beef jerky and gluten-free snacks that are not loaded with sugar. For road trips, bring a small cooler with hard-boiled eggs, chicken breast, or a dried smoothie package to which you can add water, almond, or rice milk. These are available in individual containers.

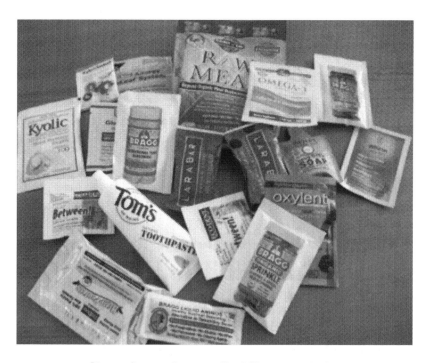

Photo of some of my goodies I like to travel with!

Healing Power of Food: Nine Excellent Food Choices so You Will Never Spend a Fortune on Medical Bills!

Did you ever stop to taste a carrot? Not just eat it, but taste it?
You can't taste the beauty and energy of the earth in a Twinkie.
~ Astrid Alauda

The Healthy Conscious Traveler will choose the following foods as often as possible when traveling. Finding organic and GMO-free food is not always easy, but do your best to honor your body.

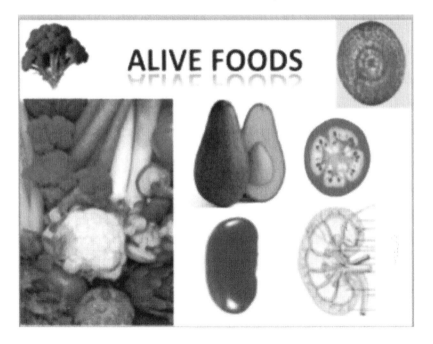

1. Greens, greens and more greens. Nutrition from nature, there is nothing better! Start each day with your favorite green smoothie and be sure to get at least three green servings per day. For lunch and dinner, add a cup of steamed or raw broccoli, asparagus, spin-ach, kale or other favorite vegetable. It's best to have fresh, but don't be afraid to prepare ahead and put in a cool container for travel. Vegetables from the cruciferous family, like kale, broccoli and cauliflower, contain powerful detoxifying compounds that protect us against environmental toxins. You will receive unbelievable results with a living foods diet, including increased energy and great moods. This is easier to do with travel than you think. Buy your favorite green drink powder, pack it in your suitcase, add water and enjoy.

A Word of Caution: Parasites can hang out in salad bars and green salad mixes, so you may just want to avoid raw salads from salad bars altogether while traveling and anytime, for that matter. Remember to always pack your digestive enzymes with hydrochloric acid for proper digestion and to protect yourself from parasites and other bugs.

2. Color your salads with vegetables that are full of carotenoids and phytonutrients, such as yellow and green zucchini, tomatoes, purple onions and cabbage, scallions and turnips. The more variety you have in your food choices, the better chance that you will consume a meal full of cell-loving nutrients and minerals. It is true, finding fresh organic salads is not always easy, but do your best to research the options before you leave. Don't be afraid to ask about the produce at restaurants. You would be surprised by what they will reveal to you, which will often help you make a quick decision.

Remember, your cells are as healthy as the food you consume, the thoughts you think, the quality of water you drink, your level of fitness and your awareness. In an interview, Mike Adams, the Health Ranger, said that "the behavior of people in a population is based on their mental health and their mental health is based on their physical health and their physical health is based on what they eat."

3. Healthy fish choices include wild fish, not farm-raised, that is fresh and low in mercury and other heavy metals. It is a great choice for your overall health. Small fish, such as sardines and scallops, tend to be lower in heavy metals because they have shorter lives and thus have a shorter time to build up toxicity. Wild fish is full of omega-3 fatty acids that are particularly good for every cell in your body. They assist with proper brain functioning and are excellent for reducing inflammation in your body. The American Heart Association recommends eating fish two to three times per week.(4) It is best to bake, broil or steam your favorite fish. Grilled fish can be carcinogenic due to the grilling process, and fried fish is often full of bad fats and loaded with calories. Top fish choices are white fish, sardines, salmon, trout and snapper. Swordfish, tuna and sea bass often have high levels of mercury.

If you are a sardine and tuna-lover like me, buy several cans of the healthiest choices, like low-mercury tuna and sardines by Vital Choice (www.vitalchoice.com/HealthyTraveler to get the Healthy Conscious Traveler special), which is also low in sodium and has no added chemicals. They are easy to pack in your suitcase and a great option for protein, when needed quickly. No matter where I go, from the bush of Kenya to the highlands of Peru or the farmlands of Haiti, I am never without my sardines, salmon or tuna and even salmon jerky! Do be aware of the potential radiation now found in some seafood from the Pacific, as a result of the Fukushima disaster.

4. Nuts and seeds are an excellent source of healthy protein, fat, fiber and minerals and a perfect choice for travel. Try organic flax, chia, raw shelled hemp seeds and pumpkin seeds (great source of zinc), as well as almonds and cashews. Fiber helps you to feel full while preventing obesity and keeps your blood sugar in balance. Fiber also reduces the risk of colon cancer and other cancers by one third. You should aim for 30 to 50 grams of fiber each day.

5. Organic grass-fed meat and farm-raised eggs are excellent choices because they are loaded with protein, iron, amino acids and omega-3s. Both these sources of protein have the power to satiate, and if you eat them on a regular basis, you can reduce your sugar cravings.

6. Consume medicinal essential oils, such as basil, lemon, clove, oregano and coriander (see Chapter 10). I bet you'll be interested in investing in the Self-care Revolution essential oils for travelers. I love starting my day with water, organic lemon juice and a hit of cayenne pepper, but while traveling I use a couple drops of lemon oil. This is a great way to detox and alkalinize your body.

7. Consume organic, quality-brand green teas, which have anti-oxidant and anti-inflammatory properties. Green herbal teas are the most widely consumed teas in the world and contain high amounts of polyphenols, which are a major factor in your longevity and will contribute to a strong heart and organ health. Check out the *Healthy Conscious Traveler's Food Guide* for great tea recipes at www.robyn benson.com.

8. Consume foods that promote healthy gut flora, such as traditionally fermented foods like sauerkraut, kefir and pickled vegetables. One of the HCT's primary goals is to maintain healthy gut flora, because this will help prevent chronic conditions and will be your best defense against all illnesses, even diarrhea, parasites and other bacterial and fungal infections. You might also consider packing blister-packed probiotic supplements that do not require refrigeration.

9. Add good fats to your diet like avocados, organic, unrefined extra virgin coconut oil and organic, extra virgin olive oil. These are necessary for your brain and cell health and can even affect the quality of your moods.

Excellent advice: *Chew more, eat less*, states the old Swedish proverb, and savor each bite. Feel the food nourish your every cell.

Bonus considerations: Take concrete steps to implement your plan of action in order to achieve your desired health goals while traveling.

Salt: Celtic or Himalayan sea salt is best. Do take a small bag or shaker for your travel meals. When dining out, ask for low or no-salt foods so you can add your own.

Water: Keep track of your daily water intake, which is so important when you travel. Rule of thumb: drink half your bodyweight in ounces of water each day. For example, a 160-pound man would need to consume 80 ounces of water. In warmer climates and with extra exertion, you might want to increase your water consumption beyond this suggestion. What is most important, however, is not always the quantity of water you drink but making sure you are absorbing the water you drink into your cells. In all cases, to better absorb water more efficiently, consider putting a tiny pinch of sea salt in your water or add Cell Food, Oxylent or other liquid trace minerals, which you can purchase in most health food stores. You will learn more about quality drinking water in Chapter 4.

Sea vegetables: There are many types of edible seaweed, often called sea vegetables as compared to land vegetables such as carrots or broccoli. Kelp, hijiki, sea palm, arame, dulse, wakame or nori can be unfamiliar names to the Westerner, yet Asian people have traditionally incorporated sea vegetables into their diet for thousands of years. Sea vegetables are an excellent source of trace minerals, such as iodine and selenium. They can help to reduce radiation sickness in general and also specifically help the thyroid, regarding radiation. While the amount of protein may be minimal, they do contain rare amino acids that combine with other amino acids in foods like beans, to make more useable complete protein.

Sea vegetables, along with salt and miso, are in the Hall of Fame for not only reducing but eliminating the effects of radiation. How can seaweed counteract radiation? One very basic example is when the U.S. dropped the atom bomb on Hiroshima and Nagasaki. Near the epicenter there was a hospital that was already providing daily miso soup with seaweed. It turned out that none of those patients in that hospital died. There was another hospital equally distant from the epicenter. Those patients, who did not have miso soup with seaweed, died – amazing and true! Canadian researchers have found a polysaccharide in seaweed that binds radioactive strontium and helps eliminate it from the body. I eat one-half sheet of nori seaweed before and after going through the airport X-ray scanner when I travel.

Food labels: Decide to make it a lifelong habit to read ingredient labels on foods and fresh produce. Beware of all food additives, food coloring and notice levels of sugar, salt and fat in your favorite foods. If the label says, "hydrogenated oils," stay away from it. It takes 50 days for the body to break down hydrogenated fatty foods, and in the meantime it creates inflammation.

Produce labeling: Have you ever wondered what the numerical labels on fruit and vegetables mean?

If the numbers begin with:

9 = Organic (enjoy without limitation)

8 = Genetically modified (run away fast!)

3 and 4 = Conventionally-grown with the use of pesticides (strictly limit your consumption)

PLEASE SHARE WITH FAMILY AND FRIENDS!

I can tell you honestly that, while traveling, other than at a spa-type accommodation, I have never seen fruits for sale that are organic in airport stores or convenience stores. Most of the produce sold in these stores are conventionally grown. Again, plan ahead and pack enough organic fruits and vegetables to last a few days when traveling domestically.

Check out www.yelp.com for consumer comments or ask your hotel concierge to direct you to the closest health food stores, farmers markets, organic restaurants, spas, hotels and gyms.

Since the US government prevents the labeling of most GMO foods, it is imperative to educate yourself on what they are and to help spread awareness. First and foremost, *avoid processed food*, and instead consume foods that are labeled USDA 100% Organic. The late fitness and food expert Jack Lalanne's motto is a good rule to live by—if man made it or altered it in any way, don't eat it!

Restaurants and Travel

I'm not against profit, but I am against negligence and the
general non-caring attitude of many of today's food (and other)
businesses. The food industry has gotten too big to be able to
be careful and conscious about the food they're growing.
~ Mark Hyman M.D.

No matter where you travel in the U.S., try to find a nearby health food store. These days, some of the larger food chains carry organic produce and goods. In Cabo San Lucas, Mexico, my girlfriends and I were excited to find a clean, well-stocked health food store close to our hotel. As consumers make their needs known, finding healthy organic foods away from home will become more common.

Be careful of franchise restaurants and any restaurant that serves factory-made, pre-prepared entrees. Most prepared food is loaded with chemicals and preservatives. There are a few franchise exceptions that provide some healthy foods like Chipotle, Noodles & Company, Cosi, Panera and Au Bon Pain. Some other franchises are also starting to offer healthier choices. If possible, eat at locally owned restaurants that use healthy local produce in meals that are cooked from scratch. Restaurant owners who do this will be proud to let you know!

For short trips of less than three days, consider purchasing frozen, delicious and healthy meals. You can pack them frozen and enjoy when you get to your destination. I have had no issue with getting assistance at any travel destination to have a meal heated up for me. I feel better knowing the source of my food.

I am happy to share that I have discovered a ridiculously convenient, healthy solution: Artisan Bistro! To learn more or to order, go to www.robynbenson.com Practitioner Code **126178**.

Artisan Bistro partnered with a group of leading practitioners to create a menu that uses proven, effective weight management research. These meals ignite your metabolism and only use the best, all-natural, organic and sustainable ingredients.

- Delicious Pre-Prepared Meals
- Wild-Caught Fish and Free-Range Meats
- Natural, Organic and Sustainable Ingredients
- GMO Free
- Gluten & Peanut Free
- Soy & Dairy Free Options
- Delivered Right to Your Door

Allergies and Gut Inflammation

Your gut is the seat of your immune system. When your gut is com-promised, often by poor dietary choices, it can create tiny pockets or gaps in your intestinal wall. This process allows substances such as undigested food, bacteria and metabolic wastes, which should be confined to your digestive tract, to escape into your bloodstream. This condition is called Leaky Gut Syndrome, and it can lead to all kinds of health issues, from headaches to gastric upset and joint pain. Once the integrity of your intestinal lining is adversely af-fected and there is a flow of toxic substances "leaking" out into your bloodstream, your body experiences significant increases in inflammation.

Dr. Robynne K. Chutkan, founder and medical director of Georgetown University Hospital's Digestive Center for Women, says: "Leaky gut can be a difficult diagnosis to establish for a num-ber of reasons: it's associated with a wide range of seemingly un-connected symptoms; it has a lot of different causes; there's no specific test to confirm it; and evidence tying it to other conditions can be murky. As a result, there's a fair amount of skepticism in the mainstream medical community about the legitimacy of leaky gut as a diagnosis. But as the evidence that this is indeed a real and recognizable condition grows, opinions are slowly changing. That's a good thing, because leaky gut is likely to emerge as one of the most significant medical concepts of our time."(5)

It would be in your best interest (to avoid or stop perpetuating leaky gut) to work with your health provider to determine your food sensitivities and other factors that may be affecting your digestive health. There are, typically, delayed food reactions that can occur over a period of seventy-two hours after consumption of the of-fending food. Acute food allergies tend to be a more sudden type of reaction; for example, the common peanut allergy can cause a serious and even life-threatening response from the body's natural defense system.

Visit your local allergy specialist for allergy testing. Otherwise, there is a reasonably priced skin prick test that will help you learn if you are sensitive to any of almost a hundred different foods. I highly recommend this test to the traveler with frequent diges-tive problems, sinus infections and a susceptibility to hives and skin rashes. As you may know, allergies are becoming more com-mon among people worldwide. See Chapter 10 for laboratory test recommendations.

Annual blood tests are advised for all HCTs

Make sure to get an annual blood test to determine the status of your immune system, as well as your adrenal, thyroid and liver function, your blood sugar levels and vitamin D levels, to name just a few of the possible options. I also highly recommend a hormone panel (blood or urine), as it will help identify levels of cortisol, the stress hormone marker and determine how well your hormones are functioning. Identifying any imbalance in your hormones and cor-recting them can be life changing.

Request the following tests:

- Chemical screen/HDL/CBC
- Thyroid panel (complete with TSH, Free T3 and Free T4)
- Insulin levels
- Hemoglobin A1C
- Homocysteine and C-reactive protein (to determine your inflammation levels)
- Vitamin D3 level- 25(OH)D

Also consider:

- Celiac panel
- Food sensitivity test
- Heavy metal testing (including blood mercury and lead levels)
- Stool, blood, urine and saliva tests for hormones, parasites and fungus, etc.

Any body dysfunction, be it physical, mental, or emotional, is a direct result of a type of deficiency for which the body can no longer cope or find ways to compensate. Certain blood tests, stool tests and saliva tests can reveal an excess of bacteria, parasites, fungus, or a hormone imbalance. By working with a holistic, integrative doctor, you can find exactly what you need to **regain and renew** your life by supplementing with what you exactly need and also by getting rid of what is not welcome in your body. These lingering pathogens can wreak havoc in your body by depleting your energy and your immunity. By making the commitment to achieve excellent health, it is important that the HCT be aware of the usefulness of these tests in diagnosing possible health conditions.

Rather than giving my patients 20 different random supplements, I do a thorough blood test evaluation to reveal the deficiencies in their bodies. Remember that diseases are often related to a lack of vitamins, minerals, amino acids, water, relaxation, even love and touch—and don't forget the most important vitamin of all: the earth's frequencies. I call those frequencies Vitamin E for Earthing or Vitamin G for Grounding.

If you suffer from depression, anxiety, or other mood disorders, know that these can also be caused by deficiencies of essential vitamins such as folate, Vitamin D3, B6, minerals, such as magnesium, zinc, selenium and lithium, amino acids and fatty acids and NOT a deficiency of Prozac, Paxil, or Zoloft or any other popular pharmaceutical drugs used for these conditions! High levels of mercury, lead, cadmium, aluminum and other heavy metals in our body also wreak havoc on our biology and contribute to our bad moods and depressed nation. I recommend that you get a heavy metal assessment from your doctor, and the lab I recommend can be found in the Resource section in Chapter 10.

For more information about supportive herbs and supplements for your travel experience, please refer to Chapter 9. In addition, see Chapter 10 for a variety of resources for your optimal health, at home or while traveling.

Call to action:

- Are you ready to grasp the information you gained from this chapter and to test your Healthy Conscious Traveler's IQ? If so, take the test in Appendix A and you'll be a Healthy Conscious Traveler for all your journeys to come.

- I invite you, your family and your friends to be part of the online free, Self-care Revolution series www.jointheselfcare revolution.com and the www.healthytravelerssummit.com.

- Promote a world without chronic diseases by following The HCT 8 Pathways. Start a food journal today. Do some detective work by jotting down everything you consume each day for a week. Make note of how you feel when you eat certain foods. Is your mood and energy better or worse after you eat?

- Favor a plant-based diet, even while traveling. Decide before you travel to eat at least 90% real food. My friend Sean Croxton, founder of Underground Wellness Channel, created the acronym "JERF," which stands for "Just Eat Real Food." Vote with your dollar and promote living foods in airports and convenience stores. That would include more organic fruits and vegetables with biodegradable forks, knives, spoons and wrapping.

- Support tax incentives for businesses that are providing healthy and eco-friendly products, foods and services.

- Download the app ShopNoGMO from the Institute of Responsible Technology on your smartphone to learn about the impact of GMO foods on your health and find the list of safe Non-GMO foods, including the Dine Out Non-GMO list.

- For current health information visit my blog: <u>robyn benson.com/blog</u>. My favorite health blogs are listed in the Resource section in Chapter 10.

Chapter 3

Exercise and "Earthing" to Enhance Your Travel Experience

When health is absent, wisdom cannot reveal itself, art cannot manifest, strength cannot fight, wealth becomes useless and intelligence cannot be applied. ~ Herophilus

Movement is a medicine for creating change in a person's physical, emotional and mental states. ~ Carol Welch

Those who think they have not time for bodily exercise will sooner or later have to find time for illness. ~ Edward Stanley

Travel, Health and Fitness

You have the potential for a long, healthy life, especially when you follow your body's natural operating instructions. In other words, you were given this amazing body that is designed to be a vibrant functioning vessel every day of your entire life.

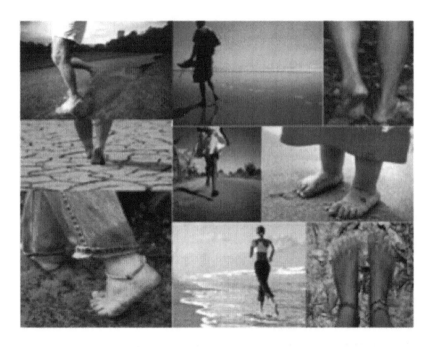

As you read further in this book, it becomes absolutely clear that the choices you make at any given time are either supporting your future destiny or taking away from your healthy blueprint. In Chapter 1, we discovered how "frequency matters" and that when you support your body with life-promoting frequencies—those found most prominently from the earth—you are bound to feel great. In Chapter 2, you learned how food is medicine and the frequency of a food either adds a good charge to your body or ultimately causes your health to deteriorate.

Exercise is also medicine for your body, mind and spirit and is yet another significant pathway for daily health. It is one of the most important ways for the HCT to achieve optimal health and to sustain radiant vitality. To ensure your beautiful destiny, free of ill health and immobility, always include exercise in the days and weeks throughout your life. Our bodies are designed for movement, and there are no exceptions.

In America today, we are lucky to walk more than two-tenths of a mile over the course of a day. Think about it: you get up, get dressed, walk to your car, walk into work, walk out of work, get back into your car and then you drive home. Perhaps you first walk through a grocery store before you go home which might add in a few hundred more steps. Can you relate to this scenario?

According to a report from the Center for Disease Control, the lack of physical activity is widespread throughout all age groups. Only about 22% of adults engage in some type of physical activity on a daily basis. Maybe only 15% to 20% routinely exercise vigorously. Nearly 50% of all youth are not active on a daily basis, and some 60% of adults do not achieve the recommended amount of regular physical activity, while 25% of all adults are totally inactive.

Regular exercise is uncommon in the elderly, with less than 10% of this age group engaging in physical exercise. About two-thirds of elderly people are either inactive or completely sedentary. (1)

Do you fit exercise into your overfilled schedule? As an HCT you must be proud to be part of the *minority* of people who actually exercise and move their body for at least 10- 20 minutes, five times a week.

Did you know inactivity is linked to the top 10 causes of disease, and to just about any disease, including heart disease, diabetes, infectious diseases, cancer and even dementia? Inactivity is responsible for more than a quarter million deaths each year. Only smoking, which kills nearly one-half million people yearly, causes more preventable deaths. In addition to lost lives, inactivity-related illnesses cost close to $1 trillion per year.

Without a doubt, you grew up hearing about the merits of exercise. Whether you surf, golf, play tennis, take a three-hour hike in the wilderness or get up early for one of a variety of boot camp classes offered in your community, you know that moving your body is essential to a healthy daily lifestyle and is often a lot of fun, too. Why wait for a medical diagnosis or crisis to wake you up to the need for exercise? The HCT knows better, right?

Do you think our ancestors ever viewed exercise like we do today? They didn't have any other option. During hunter-gatherer days, we had no choice but to walk many miles a day to gather food and water and look for shelter. Exercise in those days was a way of life and ultimately a way to sustain life. Today, really, is no different.

Today, you might use exercise to tame your overwhelmed life, to lose weight or to manage your often compulsive and unconscious eating habits. You may exercise with the enduring desire to have well-proportioned arms and shapely thighs and bottoms. Or perhaps you exercise because you hear it is the healthy thing to do. It is through exercise that you are able to perform at higher energy levels and it can also be your way to be in the great outdoors or spend quality time with friends.

Move to Jive and Thrive as You Travel

HCT, whether you are living in the Red, Yellow or Green Zone (as shown in Chapter 1), exercise and movement are essential for your cellular health, and there are very few exceptions, no matter what your health situation is. Even if you have an autoimmune disease or a disability, it is still essential for your health to move your body. And don't forget, exercise is important to sustain a healthy sex drive and to keep that lovin' feelin' alive.

When you exercise regularly, you often feel and look better and you get the added benefit of detoxifying your body through sweating. Perspiration cleanses your lymphatic system and improves your overall health and immunity. Sweating also helps to move unwanted toxins out of your blood and circulatory system. However, when you exercise to the extreme, for example excessive aerobic exercise without rest days, you can burn out your adrenal glands and disrupt your hormones and sleep cycles. Then it is easy for your body to break down.

Regular travel can be stressful, so you want to know about a stress hormone called cortisol, which is secreted by the adrenal glands when you are under stress. It is supportive in an emergency and can give you the extra strength to endure a sudden shock to the body, but it can also quickly lift you out of a deep sleep when plagued with anxiety after receiving disturbing news.

Due to the high levels of stress most people are experiencing today, which I would call Red Zone living, cortisol is being pumped out at alarmingly high rates on a regular basis. This can lead to high levels of cortisol in the blood and eventually adrenal exhaustion, a serious condition called Addison's disease. Extreme variations in cortisol can also lead to bone loss, extra weight on your body (that dreaded muffin top), headaches, body pains and memory loss, just to name a few of the common signs and symptoms.

In an interview for the Self-care Revolution, Dr. Sara Gottfried, a Harvard-trained gynecologist and *New York Times* bestselling author, said it best: "Cortisol is a bad boyfriend hormone you should have never dated because it causes lots of issues to your hormonal overview."

Exercise is essential in balancing high levels of cortisol in your bloodstream and can be the best antidote to stress. Since travel is often erratic and comes with lots of twists and turns and stressful moments, being physically fit can be your best defense in navigating through these unpredictable situations. Many studies show that regular exercise helps to clear excess levels of cortisol in the body. So, never leave home without your exercise gear!

When to push and when to let go

My friend Dr. Richard Fenker, author and sports psychologist, tells me that in order to be healthy in today's world, we have to know when to push and when to let go with all activity. He says that one common theme that is a critical part of sports and exercise is intentionality. Letting go is about flow and relaxing, and this brings the balance between pushing and letting go. This balance is essential for peace of mind and to experience joy. It is often difficult to let go and to take time just to relax. On the other hand, too much pushing causes stress. The left brain pushes and the right brain lets go. "We need a balance to sustain optimal health and to achieve this we need to be intentional with our life choices." Dr. Fenker says.

When I asked Dr. Fenker how he takes care of himself with all of his travels, he answered, "It has been 25 years since I have been ill. I believe my ability to let go keeps me from getting stressed out. I am relaxed by nature and that helps, and I believe we can all maintain this state. I am playful and I exercise regularly. I use self-talk and I listen, which guides me to let go. My goal in life is to stay relaxed, find joy in everyday living and not get sick."

I meditate for 15 minutes a day and that helps keep stress, or my perception of stress, away. I recommend that everyone meditate. In terms of exercise, research of football teams shows that when the players meditated regularly, on average they had one-half of the injuries during the season. I believe this applies to all people and certainly for the seasoned traveler. If you meditate (letting go) and practice mindfulness techniques (Pathway 8) this helps you in all the movement (pushing) that happens throughout the day, so you have the opportunity to enjoy all of life, no matter where you are.

Almost everyone I interviewed for this book spoke about the efficacy of a meditation practice, and how it can be one of your best tools to ensure peace of mind while traveling, no matter what happens. It makes sense that meditation facilitates the Green Zone lifestyle. Staying in the Green Zone as much as possible should be one of your goals as an HCT.

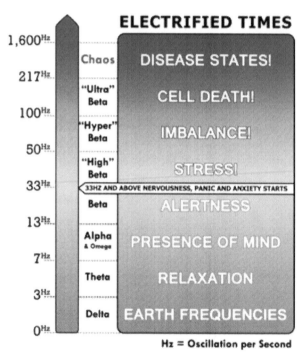

Figure 3A

Exercise Is Medicine

The most important way to get the "holy spark" of the earth's magnetic field into your cells to produce energy, known as adenosine triphosphate (ATP), is through movement. The electromagnetic field of the earth is a stagnant field, and you need to move in order to pump the earth's frequencies into your cells, thus initiating cellular health and energy. In other words, as you move you are allowing the magnetism of the earth to engage with your cells. This increases the sodium potassium pump that creates energy production through the mitochondria, the energy-producing center of the cell, in a way that allows your body systems to operate.

Remember, we are electrical beings first and foremost, and our electromagnetic balance precedes the workings of our biochemistry. Therefore, exercise plays a key role in how your metabolism works and is critical to energy production.

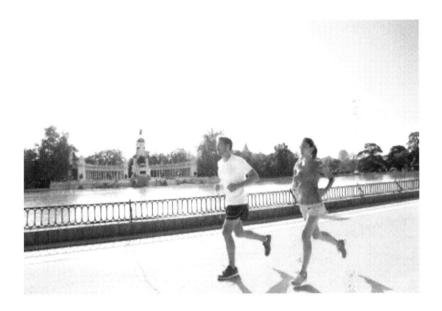

It is important that you exercise while traveling as much as possible. It is one of The 8 Pathways to travel and live healthily in this time of great change. It is certainly one of the best ways to prevent the inconvenience and expense of dealing with an illness.

Epigenetics, the study of how our environment impacts our genetics, shatters the idea that you are a victim of your inherited genes. Instead, you have tremendous power to shape and direct your physical health. Exercise, along with the right food choices, can shape your genetic future. If you eat processed foods that are foreign to the nature of your body and you lack daily movement, you can turn on genes that support a predisposition to heart disease, diabetes and other health challenges.

Truthfully, if aging were a disease, exercise, along with the other tenets of The 8 Pathways, would be your best defense against rapid decline in health and longevity. So if you are a longevity enthusiast who loves to travel, it is essential that you regularly practice all of The 8 Pathways.

Now that we understand our intimate connection to the earth, to nature and to the life-sustaining frequencies of the earth, it makes sense that exercise, in most cases, is more beneficial when it happens outdoors. When I was in China, I loved to ballroom dance outside with the Chinese people, and I even lined up in parks doing Tai Chi and Qi-Gong with my new friends. I was even brave enough to bicycle daily with all the other commuters in traffic that was worse than the streets of New York City.

Ever since I was 14, I have been an avid runner. In terms of my global travels, this has proved to be a smart habit, as I feel running has allowed me to see parts of countries that most people may never see: back alleys, early-morning prayer offerings, cobblestone roads too narrow for cars to get through.

In places like Bali, Haiti and India, I have enjoyed watching people dressed in colorful outfits as they work in the heat of the day for harvest. Tending fields and gardening are still the best forms of exercise, because you are moving as you are connecting with the soil, the minerals and the planet itself. This is one of the reasons that gardening is so popular! People love how they feel when they are digging and touching the earth and creating beauty. This is also part of the perfect formula for balancing the emotions. Because the

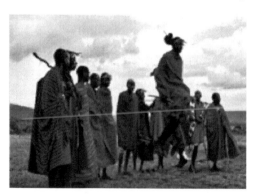

benefits of exercise do not stop at country borders, when I was in Kenya, my new tribal friends helped me realize that movement such as running, jumping, climbing and dancing are all basic to the energetic needs of their culture and for their overall health.

As I think of my travels and reflect on all that I have learned from the indigenous people of the world, I realize how much we can model after our nomadic friends to find our best approach to exercise while on the road or even in the air.

So what does this look like? You can jump in place for 10 to 30 seconds to get your heart rate up, like the Masai do. And they love to dance! Get your knees up high. Turn on your favorite music and dance in your hotel room. Take the stairs and avoid escalators. Choose to walk in most cities and avoid public transportation to get a better glimpse of daily life, wherever you may be visiting.

Essentially, there are no excuses when you consider that most of the world is inhabited by people without cars. They have no choice but to move their bodies and therefore avoid many of the diseases we are plagued with in the modern world due to lack of exercise.

Of course, only follow the above recommendations if you are in good aerobic shape. Travel is not the time to be a weekend warrior and find yourself injured. This is why the HCT works to always have an exercise routine in place throughout life.

Let's go outside

Workout in a gym or park?

What is your best choice between a workout in a gym or workout in a park? A study published in the research journal *Environmental Science & Technology* suggests that we should go for the park. Exercising outdoors not only appears to promote physical health but also boosts mental and emotional well-being. The team analyzed data from a number of sources, including eleven randomized as well as non-randomized control trials incorporating information from more than 800 adults. The study found that exercising in natural environments decreases feelings of tension, confusion, anger and depression, while increasing feelings of joy, energy levels, and engaging with others. People who exercise outdoors also are more likely to increase their exercise activity because of these benefits. (2)

Gyms around the globe are notoriously busy around the New Year with people inspired by New Year's resolutions. By March, most of these people have dropped away from the gym, while the trails are full of people hiking and the parks are abuzz with children and families in physical activities. Also, it's rare to see an empty beach in the warmer months. People crave outdoor life, but the big question is how to carve out time in your daily life so that you can be outdoors more often, moving and breathing in the fresh air?

As the HCT, outdoor exercise is not always possible with early morning flights, or with the severe air pollution that is often found in and around airports. Breathing in fumes from buses and the exhaust of automobiles and chemicals from jet fuels can be detrimental, so in this case, I recommend indoor exercise. Fortunately, many airport hotels have well-equipped fitness rooms for your exercise needs. With such a wide variety of choices from treadmills to elliptical machines and free weights, even fitting in 20 to 30 minutes would benefit your overall health, and in most cases, calm your nerves and mind.

Do your best to make time for at least 10 minutes of High Intensity Interval Training (HIIT), and don't forget to do a short warm up before and cool-down after you're done. HIIT is exercise that occurs in faster bursts (30 to 60 seconds) to get your heart rate up followed by rest (90 to 120 seconds). This is one of the best overall fitness regimens recommended by many fitness gurus today. Do seek counsel to avoid unnecessary injuries.

Good news! San Francisco International Airport is the first airport in the U.S. to open up a yoga/exercise studio, followed by the Dallas-Fort Worth Airport, which also has a yoga studio. On my way through Dallas, I came across such a place and met a wonderful therapist who helped me de-stress and relax. This kind of travel service is ideal for long layovers. Let's hope other airports catch on soon! For more information on airports that support your fitness, art and relaxation interests, view http://stuckattheairport.com.

I look forward to the day when there are medical spas in all airports with oxygen bars, IV therapies, and pulsed electromagnetic field (PEMF) mats. How about a back massage or a 30-minute acupuncture session and/or chiropractic treatment for your travel-worn body? It might be a bit out of your way but the Dubai Airport offers a 24-hour gym with private showers and steam rooms, saunas and jacuzzis. Swedish and shiatsu massages are also available while you are waiting for your next flight.

I would love to have the opportunity to stock my travel kits in these airport spas along with my top 20 herbal and vitamin formulas! I see the idea of the travel airport spa exploding in the near future, as more HCT's are traveling and making this request.

What Is Your Exercise Personality?

Do you prefer cardiovascular workouts: weight training, slow yoga stretches or CrossFit workouts that are a combination of high-intensity cardio and resistance training? Based on my research, most people seem to have an inclination for certain exercises; yet the common belief these days is to mix up your exercise routine with various types of exercises. You also need to determine which current fitness craze is worth your money, energy and time, especially with travel. Remember, get professional training where appropriate to avoid all injuries.

Top recommendations from exercise experts

Let's hear what some exercise experts have to say about travel and fitness in personal interviews conducted by me.

Mark Gurule, fitness trainer and owner of New Mexico Sports and Fitness in Santa Fe, New Mexico shares the simple mission statement, "Exercise is fun," a motto that he lives by. He asks all of his clients, "What has worked for you in the past? What is most enjoyable?" He calls his fitness program *For the Fun of FIT*! He knows that to be successful with exercise, you have to be consistent and it has to become a way of life. It doesn't all have to happen in the gym. Even 15 to 20 minutes spent doing something like yard work counts in a fitness program. To stay fit while traveling, you have to be active. Often you can find a facility in the locale where you are staying. You can also carry resistance bands for a quick workout. Even a 10- to 15-minute brisk walk can deliver good cardiovascular exercise.

The seasoned HCT does not worry about gaining an extra five pounds while away. You should be able to enjoy your vacation without regret. Mark says you can choose healthy meals at least 70% of the time and the other 30%, you can indulge! "It might be 80% / 20% or 70% / 30% depending on the type of vacation," says Gurule.

For long flights, Mark recommends a series of exercises using simple stretches for ankle and calf mobility while aboard your flight. Do circle rolls often with your ankles and get up once per hour to move your hips when sitting for extended periods of time. As soon as you get off the plane, do a few minutes of stretching while you wait for your luggage or when taking a break from car travel.

Your hotel room can become your gym. Hotel rooms have so many props that are available to use for a workout. You can use chairs or even the edge of the bed and do squats to strengthen your triceps. Try simply putting your hands on the edge of the bed or the seat of a chair, face pointing away, and push up. This is great for strengthening your triceps. It's a great idea to travel with resistance tubes with handles. You can find them at any sporting goods store. Just remember to pack them in your suitcase. Mark says, "Self-care is not the responsibility of your insurance company or your doctor, it is yours!"

Del Miller, Ph.D., founder of the *Best You Academy*, says, "Exercise does not have to be a time zapper and take hours out of your travel days." He has a formula for transforming your life and becoming fit in just 10 minutes a day. In a recent interview, he discussed how 10-minute workout sessions, including fast working and short burst sessions, can radically change the quality of your life. He asks each of us, "Would you choose your body to live in? If not, get moving!"

Keira Newton, owner of DKB fitness, a Kettlebell fitness center in Santa Fe, New Mexico, and one of my favorite places to exercise, gives us her best recommendation for the frequent flier and traveler. She believes it is essential to develop the muscles in your core abdominal area, the center around which all other muscles in your body operate. A simple exercise to build core is the "plank," which is an exercise that looks like a push-up, where your forearms rest on the floor while your legs are extended behind you. Hold for at least 20 to 30 thirty seconds, rest, and repeat. With core strength you can

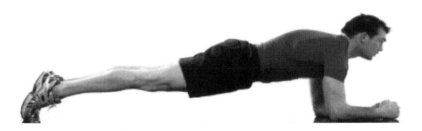

rest assured, knowing that you will be more fit and able to endure the twists and turns of travel, from lifting suitcases to endless walking on city streets or dancing the night away.

Levi Ben-Shmuel, *Huffington Post* contributor and movement enthusiast, recommends Sulam Chi: A Dance of Life. He says, "Be more in the flow of life through the gentle, simple, and powerful Tai Chi and Kabbalah-inspired movements of Sulam Chi." This devotional exercise combines the Tree of Life and Tai Chi and incorporates a move called the Spinal Twist. With focus and relaxed breathing, this exercise provides a great way to get into your body, align your mind with your movements and let your spirit flow. Levi says, "You don't have to be a performer or an athlete to be in the flow of life."

Lorin Parrish, founder of BODY, a boutique spa in Santa Fe, New Mexico, says, "Choose an exercise program that you love, that connects you with your community of friends and that gives you the physical results you desire." She also discussed the evolution of the new athlete, including Olympic athletes. They often eat gluten-free, are open to holistic principles and know the benefits of being connected to the body of the earth.

Jini Cicero, a Los Angeles celebrity fitness trainer who draws on exercise forms from Pilates to powerlifting, says, "With exercise, to do or not to do, is not an option. Exercise is medicine, so make it a way of life for you today!" Of course, optimal nutrition, deep, regenerating sleep and stress reduction are all important parts of the picture. She urges her clients to do small bouts of exercise a few times a day, between commercials and during work breaks. Do squat jumps, push-ups, burst or interval and all-out running, as fast as possible. "You will burn more calories, too, while on the road!" says Jini.

Ray Kurshals, of Pilates Santa Fe, has been an Olympic coach, massage therapist, clinical nutritionist and extensive traveler. Kurshals says that Pilates "can be learned and practiced as a form of movement and exercise that you can practice anywhere in the world." He adds, "Pilates is about increasing and sustaining core strength which is essential to not only how you move but to prevent you from falling, while allowing energy to flow throughout your body without resistance."

A final note from Dr. Frank Shallenberger, who is a world-renowned Integrative medical doctor. He believes that a good physician needs to find the root cause of disease and not just treat symptoms. He also looks at the interactions of the different parts of the body and how they affect each other. Additionally, he believes it is essential to optimize one's oxygen utilization to feel good and avoid sickness. He agrees that we are as healthy as our 75 trillion cells, and exercise and eating healthy foods are the best ways to increase our oxygen utilization in order to keep our bodies well.

10 of the best exercises for high-performance travel on the road

Walking. There are no excuses here. Consider walking in malls and parks or up and down stairs in any hotel in which you may be staying. Walking is a great way to do moderate-intensity physical activity, which means working hard enough to raise your heart rate and break a sweat. You should still be able to carry on a conversation. For more information on everything you might want to know about walking, visit Wendy Bumgardner at www.walkingabout.com or one of the many other walking sites on the web.

Yoga. The yogic prescription for health is always do-able on the road. Be sure to download apps of yoga practices that inspire you or remember sequences that you have used before. Yoga is an excellent way to keep yourself fit and flexible while traveling. You can move and stretch in most places. Of course, you can choose to join yoga retreats around the world too. My friend Marcia Wieder, CEO of Dream University and a frequent traveler, told me about *Escape to Shape*, which offers travel and cultural connections with fitness and wellness, including daily yoga and exercise classes. Sounds like a great way to get in shape and unwind from your busy lifestyle while traveling. Visit www.escapetoshape.com.

Tai Chi and Qi-Gong are two Asian exercises practiced for both mind and body benefits and the most common forms of exercise that enhance immune, organ and brain health. For six weeks straight when I was in China, each morning I gathered with others in parks, soccer fields and tea gardens and practiced Tai Chi and Qi-Gong. Both are great for the traveler because you can practice almost anytime and anywhere. To get started now, visit my friend Allan Ting's website at http://sparkstofire.com/get-more-energy-with-allan-ting/. He will show you how to get an abundance of energy through yoga and Qi-Gong and the secrets of high-performance energy for your busy professional life.

Pilates improves flexibility, builds strength and develops control and endurance in the whole human body, according to information from the Mayo Clinic. It puts emphasis on alignment, breathing, developing a strong "powerhouse" and improving coordination and balance. (3) According to Joseph Pilates, originator of Pilates, the "powerhouse" is the center of the body, and if strengthened, offers a solid foundation for any movement. This type of exercise is offered in levels from beginning to advanced.

Running and swimming. Choose one of these cardiovascular exercises that you love, and aim for 20 minutes three to four times a week. Maybe it is swimming or water aerobics that you enjoy. Fortunately, there are pools in hotels and local communities worldwide. My favorite place to swim is in the ocean, and I love to run on the beach, especially barefoot. To me this is the ultimate way to connect to the healing properties of the earth (earthing).

High-intensity or High-intensity Interval Training (HIIT) is a 10- to 20-minute burst workout for those who are fit. Consider adding three high-intensity workouts to your weekly menu, especially if you're wanting to lose fat. Although there are many programs to choose from, this is the one I value: It includes a warm up/cool down for five minutes (run, bike, swim, etc.), followed by 30 seconds of a quick burst, a rest for 90 seconds, then 30 seconds fast. Repeat this sequence eight times.

Weight Lifting. Healthy bones and tissue require strength training. Two to three times a week, use resistance bands, dumbbells, kettlebells or use your own weight (use a bench behind you and lift your body weight with your arms). Make sure you get proper training from a certified fitness trainer.

Zumba and **Nia Dance** classes are now available all around the country and internationally too. Trust me, you will feel better in your body after a class like this. This is self-healing through the joy of movement, while enjoying eclectic and sensual music from around the world.

CrossFit Gyms (www.crossfit.com). This type of exercise, developed by Coach Greg Glassman over several decades, offers constantly varied movements performed at high intensity. It has a communal aspect, meaning that there is community that arises spontaneously when people do these workouts together. Like Kettlebell, begin by taking a fundamentals class.

Put your hotel room to work. This is another great habit to commit to while on the road. Roll out of bed into your makeshift exercise room. It may sound ridiculous, but you can get the best workouts ever in your hotel room. I sure do, while being careful not to impact the people on lower floors. Here is a great invigorating hotel workout I use. This may seem repetitious, but in the words of the infamous Tony Robbins, repetition is the mother of skill. The HCT lives by design, not default, so we want to make sure you have not missed a beat here.

Hotel Room Exercise: Only do these exercises if you are fit and your doctor has cleared you:

- Jump rope x 100 (always keep one in your suitcase)
- Run in place for 3 to 5 minutes (if vigorous 1 minute then take a break)
- Jumping jacks x 100 (10 x 10) is fine too
- Knee lifts 10 x 10 and break as needed
- Sit-ups x 100
- Push-ups x 10 or your comfort zone
- Squats x 50
- Plank x 1 minute
- Run up and walk down stairs
- Yoga and or Tai Chi moves
- Join our private Healthy Traveler's Facebook page and add your suggestions: https://www.facebook.com/groups/1422321751413251/.
- See my video on my website for more about these 10 steps above.

Call to Action:

- **Stop looking for the quick fix for fitness** and avoid being a weekend warrior, which can result in injury and unhappy travel moments. If your physician has not cleared you for independent physical activity, you can exercise under the supervision of a certified professional. Yes, you can find exercise professionals in most places globally, so do your research, and get yourself an appointment before you arrive.

- **Prioritize exercise into your life** at least four times a week. Decide what your exercise personality is and mix your exercise choices for better overall fitness. For example, on your first day of travel, take a 15- to 20-minute walk to get acclimated to your new destination. Then on day two, go on a vigorous hike followed by a day of easy walking or yoga.

- Allow and plan for fitness success one day at a time. Say "yes" to exercise and cultivate the beliefs that Mark Gurule shared above, "Exercise is my medicine of choice" and "Exercise is Fun," by finding the ways you love to move.

- **Strive to go barefoot** (Earthing) and get outdoors as much as possible while on the road. Reconnect to the earth frequencies and remember the "Gushing Spring" point at the bottom of your feet that craves the earth. If possible, make sure you go to the beach at least a few times a year.

- If access to nature is not available to you nearby or even outside your door, consider lying on your favorite PEMF device (discussed in Chapter 10) that mimics nature. This is easy to travel with, as I traveled with mine to 17 countries. Honestly, in today's electro-smog world, you may find you cannot live without this wellness device to recharge your cells and to sustain daily wellness. You can go to www.join-theselfcarerevolution.com/deep-healing-frequencies/ to learn more about this excellent product.

- **Work with your fitness trainer** and ask for an exercise prescription for your travel dates. It is best to find a fitness practice that suits your health, fitness level and is fun. This is key. With so many choices these days, find a few exercise options that you actually look forward to and show up for at least four times a week.

- **What small changes will you make** to add exercise into your healthy travel blueprint? Don't allow travel to be an excuse to gain weight. For example, try setting your alarm to go off twenty minutes earlier so that you can fit movement into your new day. In the words of Dr. Alan Christianson, ND, "Commit today to 'heroic consistency' with your optimal food choices, exercise routines and value your rest time too."(4)

- **Write down your exercise schedule** for each trip you take and remember, "live by design not default." For many high-performing business people, this regular exercise routine will ensure mastery at all levels, especially when you have to give a lecture.

- **Advocate to the airport presidents and CEOs** that they consider creating exercise areas outside, around their buildings as well as in terminal areas and on rooftops. They should also take steps to greening the inside of buildings, like many European airports have done, including Amsterdam Airport Schiphol.

- **Search** www.yelp.com and www.traveladviser.com to find highly recommended gyms and other workout facilities (tennis, golf, swimming).

- **Check out** http://exerciseismedicine.org to keep up on what is available to support your exercise needs.

- **"Self-care is a way of life not an event"** is a guiding principle at my center, Santa Fe Soul Center for Optimal Health, www.santafesoul.com. It ensures a good and robust life. What three forms of movement will you commit to with each trip?

Chapter 4

Pure Water and Minerals — The Key to Your Cellular Health

Water is the only drink for a wise man. ~ Henry David Thoreau

Water is revered around the world. We are dependent on water; we can't live without it. In our mother's womb, we are nurtured for nine months in amniotic fluid, within a sacred sac of water. Many of us are baptized with water, and from the time we are conceived to the day we die, we have a symbiotic relationship with water. Thus, as a social and cultural construct, we must begin to not only recognize our innate connection and relationship with water, but we must take significant steps to protect and revere this sacred and most precious natural resource.

We need to consider water not only from a biological perspective but also from a cultural and ancestral one. Traveling the world, I have been inspired by how the people of certain cultures are in absolute awe of water, and how they value and bless every drop they drink. In my two trips to Peru, I visited Tampon, also known as *The Temple of Water* (as shown below). Just like their ancestors have done for centuries, the Peruvians still come to Tampon as a daily pilgrimage and gather water to show their respect and gratitude for this essential element on which all of life depends.

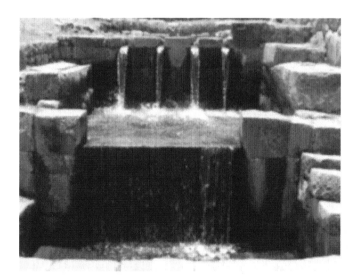

Rivers are considered by many cultures to be the veins of the earth where the blood, as water, flows. This is exactly what is happening in your body as water-rich blood is carried through your veins. We now know that we are bio-identical to the earth and what is good for the earth is also good for us.

Even though a pure water source is a human right, much of the world is living without a healthy water supply. Due to global pollution, waste dumping and mining in many countries, water is the carrier of many microbes and diseases. Probably second to breathing in oxygen, nothing is more important to the functioning and health of our bodies than pure water.

When I was in Kenya with a group of people, I was struck by all the children running towards us asking for water, not food. As we drove through the streets, children with round bellies ran up to our car asking for this most precious life-supporting liquid. The depth of our collective pain was palpable as we slowly moved from town to town, seeing the desperation in these dear faces. Human beings can live without food for awhile, but not water. Cherish the water you have on your travels.

When I was in Haiti, after the rooster's crow had awakened me, I would take early morning walks. Women and children were busy gathering water from the wells, often walking great distances back to their homes. They carried buckets of water on their heads and hips, embracing this precious liquid like a beloved child. It was painful for me as a doctor and fellow human to notice the wrinkles on the faces of the older women with loose tissue dangling from their water-deprived bodies. This scenario still goes on today. Yes, water is a human right, but much of the world still lives thirsty and without what is so important for their body's ability to thrive.

One cold March morning in Lourdes, France, I lined up with men and women to take part in the holy bath blessings. People from all over the globe came with hopes and desires for miraculous healings, such as having vision restored or being able to walk again. Others came seeking forgiveness, to be anointed with the holy water of Lourdes. One young woman standing in front of me confessed that she was there for one reason: to be blessed with a child in her womb after years of miscarriages and fertility issues. A woman, scarred from breast surgery, wailed as she slipped her body into the bath next to me, into the frigid water, with a statue of the blessed mother sitting above her.

When it was my turn, I surrendered the experience to the Divine, asking for purification on the physical, mental and emotional planes and for the strength to continue my life's calling. As I moved into the water, two women guided me on each arm. I took a deep breath, wanting to cherish each and every moment, and then sat down in the blessed water. It was freezing cold!

What is "holy water"? It's water that has been blessed and it carries a frequency, an energy of its own nature. In Fatima, Portugal, where between May and October of 1917, three shepherd children, Lucia Santos and her cousins Jacinta and Francisco Marto, reported visions of a luminous lady believed to be the Virgin Mary. The lady appeared to the children on the 13th day of each month at approximately noon, for six straight months. Fatima now attracts thousands of pilgrims from all over the world who come for healing, particularly on the pilgrimage days in May and October. I've collected water from this region and also collected water from the Chalice Well in Glastonbury, England, which is believed to possess healing properties. The well itself is thought to have been built by those of the Old Religion, the Druids, and it is claimed that the water that gushes forth from the well has magical powers.

It's no wonder that such strong convictions and intentions can result in miracles when water such as this comes in contact with the body. As we learned in the frequency flier chapter, everything is energy. When you bring intention and thought to anything (Pathway 7), the outcome can shift. If everything is energy and water carries a frequency, it follows that the waters of the world carry the frequency of humanity, as well as the animal and underworld communities.

Masaru Emoto

Dr. Masaru Emoto, who was known best for his photography of frozen water while viewed under a microscope, calls this *Hado*. He says, "I use Hado to mean all the subtle energy that exists in the universe. It is this subtle energy that carries negative or positive vibrations." Negative Hado creates incoherence and chaos, whereas positive Hado creates coherence and brilliance. As one who has traveled the world experiencing sacred water sites, I follow Dr. Emoto's suggestion that we send the Hado of peace, love and joy to bodies of water around the world, and especially to places in turmoil and war. This is something all of us who are fortunate enough to travel can do.

One Sunday afternoon a few years ago, I sat, mesmerized, in a sold-out audience at the downtown Santa Fe Lensic Theater listening to Masaru Matsumoto Emoto speak of the messages from water. He showed slides of water from Lourdes, Japan, New York City and London, just to name a few. Each slide revealed the aliveness of water, and not only how water is influenced by chemicals, but how it responds to prayers and thoughts. Some crystals looked dead and others had an effervescent, sparkly quality. I was surprised to see that New York City water and London tap water ranked higher than Los Angeles water, and even better than water from wells in some smaller towns.

Perhaps what amazed me most was learning how much our thoughts and emotions can quickly impact the sacred geometry, the resonance and overall nature and structure of water crystals. It was exciting to see that water crystals responded favorably to all spiritual traditions and their symbols. Is this another clue that there is unity in diversity?

Dr. Emoto showed that water, when placed in the energy of prayer circles, became brighter, livelier, and more resonant. Resonance is a dynamic whereby chaos in an energetic environment becomes synchronized, or more coherent. Coherence is "the quality of being logical and consistent." He showed that the higher, more resonant vibration becomes the dominant force. This is exactly what our bodies are always striving for: homeostasis, or balance. When we are living a life of balance, especially when it comes to rest, activity and how well we nourish ourselves, we tend to sustain health.

Certainly this is what each of us will strive for, "yes" resonance and coherence as we travel as an HCT through everyday life. If you are not familiar with the more than 20 years of research documented by this esteemed man, who died in October 2014, I highly recommend you Google him or visit his website.(1) Whether you are traveling or sipping water at home, his research will change how you think and feel about water.

It is wonderful to see all the organizations that are committed to creating a culture of water-conscious people, inspired by Dr. Emoto, who initiated the United Nation's declaration that the decade from 2005 to 2015 be the International Decade of Action: Water for Life. Now there is World Water Day! Emoto believed that "if children know how powerful thoughts, words and vibrations are to water, they will be able to promote the message of peace into water and into themselves starting at a young age."

The Unsinkable Dead Sea

I love trekking to sacred sites and have visited the Jordan River in Jordan and the Sea of Galilee and the Dead Sea in Israel. Each of these bodies of water have been revered as holy waters for centuries, from biblical times to the present. I spent a full day at

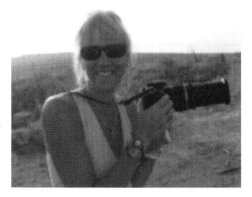

the Sea of Galilee and was able to soak my feet for hours in the Jordan River, the baptismal place of Jesus. Truly a water feast to add to my list of favorite sacred sites.

Perhaps most memorable, were my two visits to the Dead Sea in Israel where I had a blast with my friends as we put healing mud all over our bodies and faces. Mud-laden bodies were all around us, and we looked like we were all from a different planet. Due to the exfoliating and detoxifying properties, the nearby stores were stocked with this mud, complete with the promise of beautiful, youthful skin.

It was a most joyous time, floating in the Dead Sea among people from around the globe. At 400 feet below sea level, the healing properties and magical nature of this water attract people from near and far. This unsinkable water, full of rejuvenating and invigorating minerals, becomes a healing place where you can soothe aches and pains in your body, as well as having a positive effect on the emotional body. As I observed my global neighbors enjoying themselves, I simultaneously felt deeply calm and connected to the Great Spirit. I strongly encourage you to seek out sacred water sites on your travels.

Dehydration

If there is one thing I have repeated many times in my 23-year practice, it is the words "Drink more water!" Dehydration is a serious condition that can accumulate over a lifetime, eroding one's health. It is even more common when you're traveling, caused by poor hydration and eating too much sugar as well as foods full of excess sodium, chemicals and preservatives.

There is no better information on the subject of dehydration than Dr. F. Batmanghelidj's book *Your Body's Many Cries for Water.* Generally speaking, if we are listening, our bodies "speak" to us and give us signs that we need to eat and nourish ourselves. Oddly enough, from an early adult age, because of what Dr. B. calls "a gradually failing thirst sensation," we can become increasingly dehydrated without even being aware of it. This decrease in our daily water intake affects the efficiency of our cells. The ratio of water inside the cells to the volume of water outside the cells undergoes a drastic change. The loss of intracellular water creates symptoms that are often alleviated with unneeded medications by our doctors. These symptoms are often viewed by conventional medicine as part of a disease process when, in fact, the simple solution is proper hydration. Over time, chronic dehydration can cause serious damage to the human body.

One of the factors involved with dehydration, according to Dr. B., is the aging process. In effect, our bodies start out as plums and gradually become prunes. As babies we are approximately 80 to 90 percent water but as we become advanced in age we are only around 50 to 60 percent water. In a country where most people are interested in anti-aging therapies, it's a no-brainer that adequate hydration is essential for slowing down the aging process!

Less well known is that dehydration displays signs other than "dry mouth." According to a new understanding of dehydration, allergies, asthma and chronic pains could all be crisis signals of a water shortage in the body, not of injury or infection. Only water can alleviate such conditions, although conventional medical doctors may use medications or invasive diagnostic procedures instead. "Painkillers" can dull the problem, but the risk involved is that long-term dehydration, once established, can cause permanent local or general damage that may lead to an irreversible disease status.

Research reveals that some of the more common symptoms of dehydration are: dyspeptic pain, which includes gastritis, duodenitis and heartburn, aching joints, dizziness and vertigo, elevated or lowered blood pressure, muscle cramping, constipation and increased intestinal gas, scaly and dried-out skin, dark circles under the eyes and swelling/edema in the lower extremities.(2)

One of the most serious consequences of dehydration, according to Dr. Jerry Tennant in his book *Healing Is Voltage*, is that the voltage in your body becomes too low to carry on basic biological and chemical functions. To have proper water transport in and out of the cells, you need adequate levels of mineralized water. Otherwise, you may be stricken with inflammation, digestive disturbance or skin eruptions. You can easily avoid this by hydrating with well-mineralized water that ensures healthy electrical voltage throughout your cellular being.(3)

Now you know why I tell all my clients to drink more water!

Water as medicine

Water is one of the most overlooked and under-appreciated parts of the equation for optimal health. HCT, know that sustained hydration is one of the most important things you can do to thrive during your travels. It is just being conscious of this with travel in order to take care of your cells, skin and brain.

Most people are dehydrated, even people who drink a lot of water! Why? Because water that is consumed is not necessarily absorbed, due to impurities, disorganization (high surface tension) and lack of minerals. Dehydration is the root of most every known disease, and it is the reason that we may struggle with common symptoms such as headaches, constipation, acid reflux, dizziness, palpitations, wrinkled skin and hundreds of other discomforts that many experience in everyday life.

Hydration is not a common topic at your annual doctor's check-up, but my emergency room doctor colleagues agree with me that dehydration is probably the root cause of most emergency room visits, especially when traveling. The bottom line is, when you are not hydrated, your body cannot function properly.

Begin each day with two cups of room temperature water with a squeeze of organic lemon. This is one of the best ways to flush your body of toxins. Lemon juice in water alkalinizes your body and helps to awaken your electrical system, which in turn allows every organ in your body to function more efficiently. For convenience, travel with a small bottle of 100% lemon oil, and add a drop or two to your morning water.

So what exactly does water, sometimes referred to as the "elixir of life" do for you? My friend, water expert and inventor, Clayton Nolte, describes water as the quintessence or absolute embodiment of anything, a panacea and a sovereign remedy.

Our bodies are 70% water and our brain is 80 to 85% water and most cells of the body are at least 90% water. An incredible fact is that the earth is also 70% water, just like our bodies. When we consider our health, it makes sense that water is absolutely integral to our existence just as every breath we take in.

When we neglect our body's most essential needs, our system begins to break down, and the network of our body's internal systems fail to communicate efficiently. Just one day of water deprivation causes our skin to wilt, our organs to cramp, and even our brains to work less efficiently.

Another important fact about water is that it plays a very important role in our body's metabolism. Metabolism is a two-way street, involving both the breaking down of complex molecules to produce energy as well as the building up or creation of larger molecules for storage in the body. Along with food and other nutrients, water is needed for these processes, essentially sustaining our lives.

Make the choice to drink more pure water and you will experience a myriad of health benefits. When you are properly hydrated, water helps to:

- Energize your body
- Prevent depression and bad moods caused by dehydration
- Prevent water retention and bloating
- Make your skin glow
- Improve digestion
- Tone up your muscles
- Flush toxins from the body
- Increase the rate at which your liver burns fat
- Suppress your appetite
- Move blood and lymph flow through the body
- Conduct nerve impulses throughout the nervous system
- Balance hormones
- Regulate body temperature
- Regulate and cushion organs

In order for water to get inside our cells, we not only need a healthy water supply but we also need to exercise to have healthy sodium/potassium pump function that takes in water and detoxes our cells.(4) In today's world, we find ourselves stressed, rushing and always in motion but not always taking time to consciously exercise! This sodium/potassium pump is a transmembrane protein that moves sodium out of our cells and potassium into the cells. This function basically balances the relationship between sodium and potassium in our cells, keeping the cells, and thus our bodies, in balance. Keep in mind that we need movement or exercise in order for it to work.

This is not referring to the sodium in generic table salt, which lacks nutritional minerals and actually dehydrates your body. Balanced sodium and potassium are found in sea salts, such as Celtic or Himalayan salt, which are not ordinarily available to us during travel. For that reason, we need to take responsibility by bringing sea salt on our travels or a vitamin-mineral supplement you can add to water. My favorite is Oxylent, which you can find in most health food stores. The woman behind this quality supplement I use every day is Lisa Lent. Read her amazing story below.

Lisa Lent was a young flight attendant for United Airlines on an international leg from London to Washington, DC, when she suddenly felt a crushing pain in her chest. The discomfort subsided but left her concerned. Urged by her family to visit the hospital four days later, Lent was surprised to learn she had suffered a pulmonary embolism caused by several clots in her lungs. Even more surprising was what may have contributed to her condition.

She learned that low-oxygen cabin pressure, dehydration and radiation can lead to many different types of health issues. It was then she began a personal journey to create a nutritional supplement that could optimize the health of anyone from the average adult to the most vulnerable, like pregnant women and children. "My experience opened my eyes to the importance of essential nutrients and natural health and set me on a journey of healing and learning," said Lent. "It was a big wake-up call in my life that made me realize I was going in the wrong direction. I had an epiphany at that moment that I wanted to change my life."(5)

Pure water vs. processed water

We are inundated with choices when it comes to our drinking water. It is an education in itself to simply become aware of all the water options and to make informed decisions. When traveling, you won't have a lot of good choices; just use your best judgment. Ask if filtered water is available. Bottled water may not be the best, but it surely beats tap water, especially when you do not know the source of where the tap water is coming from. Glass bottles are better than plastic. When in doubt, drink boiled water.

Most people do know that tap water contains chlorine, fluoride, lead and lots of other pollutants. What many don't realize is that chlorine breaks down into chloroform in the body. Chlorine is known to be carcinogenic and especially harmful to your liver and to your brain. Chlorine is also released as a vapor when you take a hot shower. I grew up as a competitive swimmer, and I remember how sleepy I felt after swimming in a chlorinated swimming pool. Drowsiness is one of the known side effects of exposure to chlorine. Fortunately, today there are salt, ozone and freshwater systems that can be used to purify pool water.

Dr. Joseph Mercola, a leading expert in the wellness field, has released a report titled "Is Your Water Safe?" Download this free report to learn what you should know about the potential harmful effects of chlorine in your drinking water.(6)

Worldwide, water is an $80 billion business. We unwittingly contribute to the polluting of our lands as we drink from yet another plastic bottle of Fiji, Smart water or Evian (*naive* spelled backwards). Is there an ecological and economical alternative to bottled and tap water? What if planes, trains and buses were equipped with water filtering systems so that we are not contributing to the waste hazards of plastics on the earth? What if there was reverse osmosis, structured or carbon-filtered systems at airports and transportation stations? What an amazingly healthy concept!

What if airlines invested $1 to $5 of the cost of every flight in these water treatment options? Imagine water-dispensing systems in airports and planes, and all forms of transportation with water that is clean, pure, oxygenated, free of chlorine, microbes, chemicals, fluoride, pharmaceuticals, dirt, rust and heavy metals. It would be comforting to know that all the coffee, tea and other hot foods and beverages we consume at these places were made with the healthiest possible water. This can only happen if people who support the travel industry as a whole start demanding these kinds of services. This not only makes sense for the public but also for the industry employees.

Did you know that, over the past 40 years, our consumption of drinking water in plastic containers has increased by 80%? It turns out that the plastics made of polycarbonate leach the chemical bisphenol-a (BPA) into the water you're drinking. BPA, which is considered to be an endocrine disrupter, mimics estrogen and can change the way hormones function in your body. It has been linked to a range of health problems including reduced fertility, birth defects, diabetes and a higher risk of certain cancers. Unfortunately, looking for BPA-free products doesn't really solve the problem because of a similarly troubling chemical, bisphenol-S (BPS), which has been substituted for BPA in plastics due to consumer concerns. According to an article in *Scientific American*, BPS may be just as harmful as BPA.(7)(8)

Structured water

> *The more you filter water the more artificial it becomes.*
> *~ H4H (Hydration 4 Health) Initiative*

Most of us don't consume water directly from nature. There is really only one type of water that you are designed for and that is structured water, which is water directly from nature. The water in your cells is actually structured.

What is structured water? There is a life force in water that flows naturally in springs and rivers. In nature, water is filled with strings of liquid crystals. These crystals actually vibrate at a very high frequency and hold a negative electrical charge known as negative ions. This water is structured.

Did you know that healthy air and pure water are loaded with negative ions? This negative charge is necessary for water to be absorbed into your cells. Unhealthy water and air, on the other hand, give out a positive ionic charge, which means it is acidic and is less likely to be absorbed into your cells. How can we expect our cells to absorb liquid that is no longer organized in a way that communicates with our cells?

At a recent conference I attended, Dr. Edward F. Group, D.C., said, "Structured water is health in liquid form, because it delivers its gifts to us according to its Original Intention. The light, and therefore, the life in processed and treated water is greatly diminished, energetically speaking, in part because it is out of balance. It will therefore produce a dimmer 'biophotonic signature' than that of a structured water cluster. The cluster sizes are also smaller for structured water, and in this case, smaller cluster sizes and lower surface tension means easier cellular access and communication, and hence, more effective hydration." Dr. Group also states, "While there are many ways to structure water, from technological to spiritual, Clayton Nolte's technological method unifies both worlds into one."(9)

Clayton Nolte has developed the now re-named PHOTONIC water structuring device. This method, which uses no electricity, magnets or any other outside force, creates a major increase in the presence of light or bio-photons in the water. The structuring of water clears it of memory, which refers to the molecular bonds that are accumulated as it travels through the waterways to you. Structured water can improve one's inner environment or inner ecology, which has been shown to be able to restore your health and well-being.

THE HEALING PROPERTIES OF STRUCTURED WATER

At Santa Fe Soul, my health and wellness center in Santa Fe, New Mexico, our clients line up with their glass and BPA-free plastic containers to receive our structured and filtered water. Our structuring device comes from Clayton Nolte's company, Natural Actions Technologies, which uses sacred geometry in a range of products both portable and for home use. It cleanses and filters out serious waterborne microbes that have been known to wipe out herds of livestock. Once water passes through these advanced filtering and structuring systems, the water becomes "wetter" and is more easily absorbed into the cells of the body.(10)

We also have a Japanese ionized water filtration system, called Athena, which gives you the option of acidic, purified or alkaline water, and it even talks to you to let you know the choice you are making. I must say that I am not convinced that alkaline water created from these sink top devices is the way to go.

Although the technology of these water filtration systems is impressive, I believe that the best way we can get true structured and healthy water is directly from the earth, from natural springs. To find a spring near you, visit www.findaspring.com. However, due to the extreme pollution that we humans have created, the availability of these pure water sources has decreased markedly. Therefore, I carry my Natural Action Technologies hand-held portable device to filter all my beverages. It's easy to use, once I pass TSA, to drink available water, even from a drinking fountain. (See photo below!)

Eat your water

The quest for the healthiest water can be quite a journey and confusing to say the least. Organic fresh fruits and vegetables (look for the #9 code stickers) are one of the best choices for hydrating your body while traveling, as they contain naturally high-pH waters. Once again, always look to nature to solve your health concerns. Consider how satisfying and refreshing a tasty organic apple can be or how it feels to bite into a juicy, ripe, organic strawberry. This is what I refer to as eating your water and getting what nature provides naturally. Remember, water is supposed to be wet, pure and full of negative ions and free of anything nature hasn't put there originally. With organic produce, you mostly cannot go wrong.

When you eat celery, a high water content food, you are also ingesting a vegetable that not only looks like a bone, but has the exact same chemical mineral composition as bones. For example, bones consist of about 22 essential minerals, which are the same as what you consume when you eat a stalk of organic celery.

HCT, as you travel, do your best to eat your water with every meal you choose. For example, have a protein smoothie with blueberries or blackberries. For extra hydration, add structured water to get the full oxidant power of the fruit. Water from nature is easy for your cells to assimilate, and you will have much more vitality and resiliency as you move through your days of travel.

Organic, raw and fresh fruit and vegetable juices contain potent electromagnetic energy and supply extra electrons to stabilize disease-promoting free radical molecules. Fresh fruit and vegetable juices have reduced H_2O molecule size, just like real water, and contain a lower surface tension and a higher pH. Go to www.robynbenson.com to download the *Healthy Conscious Traveler's Food Guide* to find some water nourishing recipes!

Water and Environmental Concerns

The Fukushima Daiichi nuclear disaster of March 11, 2011, is adding radioactive materials into our rainwater and oceans on a daily basis. There are reports of elevated levels of radiation in many areas of California and other neighboring states and even as far away as the East Coast of the U.S.

Traveling to developing nations has its own set of issues for you, HTC, from all kinds of waterborne insects and microbes to other forms of pollution. Be careful. Always drink bottled water and pray that it is bottled properly. A seal around the cap is a positive sign.

There is also the issue of pharmaceuticals, heavy metals and other foreign toxic contaminants that are found in our water supply. The bottom line is: be prudent! Do not brush your teeth from taps in developing nations. Always ask the front desk at any hotel you travel to about the quality of their water. Is it okay to drink? Is it treated water? You have the right to know about the quality of the drinking water at public places. Also, ask these questions at all restaurants where you eat. This is why it is necessary to stay away from street vendor food in developing nations and in any country, for that matter.

Not only is the water source questionable, but also the type of oils used in cooking. If they are rancid, GMO (soy, canola and cottonseed) or have been left out in the heat and light of the day, they can be toxic to your body.

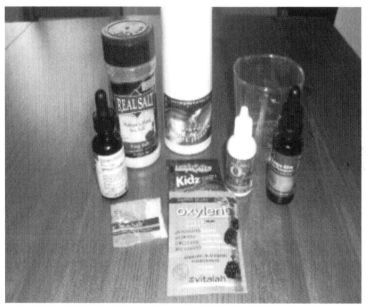

Hydration Recommendations for the HCT: Travel sea salt, Liquid Chlorophyll, Real salt, Natural Action Technologies structured water device (pour beverages through the top into your glass), Aerobic 07, Oceans Alive mineral supplement, Kids Emergence C and Oxylent

1. The number one recommendation is to eat a high-water-content diet on a regular basis, including fruits, veggies and live foods. Make sure to drink at least 48 to 64 ounces of healthy, mineralized water each day.

2. Add Aerobic O7 to your water. It is known to be effective against salmonella, cholera, E.coli, streptococcus and even against giardia lamblia. (Available at http://www.shopnhr.com/.)

3. Add liquid minerals to your water. My favorite is the brand Oxylent, an oxygenating, hydrating and rejuvenating packet you can add to water that provides enzymes, electrolytes, amino acids as well as vitamins and minerals. It does not have added sugar or preservatives. (Available at https://www.oxylent.com/.)

4. Add a pinch of sea salt in water, or put directly in your mouth followed by water to help with absorption of water into your cells. To more fully understand the electrical nature of water and the sodium-potassium pump mentioned in this chapter, check out this site: http://www.konaseasalt.com/index.php/about-kona-sea-salt/hawaii-sea-salt-and-your%20health/206.(11)

Important Highlights from This Chapter

- Water is sacred and is a human right. Bring presence and gratitude to this invaluable essential element, as there is no life without it.

- For water to be useful and to be absorbed properly into your cells, add electrolytes, including sodium and potassium.

Call to action:

- Before you travel, know your hydration plan. How will you consume a water-rich diet, and what will you do to ensure that you drink at least 48 to 64 ounces of water each day?

- Download one of a few water apps to monitor your drinking each day. Personally, I track my water consumption in my fitbit log. (See https://www.fitbit.com.)

- Bless your water and be grateful for each sip as it brings its life-supporting hydrogen, oxygen and, as Dr. Emoto says, "Hado" to your cells.

- Drink 8 to 16 ounces of clean water and 1 to 2 drops of lemon juice or lemon oil first thing in the morning. Do this as often as possible throughout your life.

- Travel with your own portable structured water device and use it with all water, coffee and even your wine, to have a constant source of clean, refreshing water and liquids. In the picture above, the tall filtering unit costs $349. This 10-ounce white plastic canister is practically indestructible. To get a special offer for the Health Travelers community, visit https://bhe88838.isrefer.com/go/specialoffer/a172/. This portable device can also be used for what is called "Structured Breathing," also known as "Qi-Gong through a tube." Do both to feel more alive, awake and more enthusiastic.

- Bring your portable filtering and structuring device on all trips and especially when camping. REI.com has quite a list of portable water-filtering devices. I also recommend Lifestraw. The LifeStraw device enables users to safely drink water from any water source, including contaminated sources. Also, they have a good cause behind the product. For every LifeStraw product purchased, a school child in a developing country is provided with safe drinking water for an entire school year. You can buy a LifeStraw water bottle at www.buylifestraw.com and use it for all your water travel needs.

- The founder of Charitywater.org shared with me the incredible effort his organization is doing to provide water to communities globally. If you are moved to do so, make a donation to www.charitywater.org. Imagine your life without access to clean running water. Imagine having to walk for *hours* each day, to fetch dirty and often disease-ridden water for your family's survival. This is how millions of our fellow human beings exist right now. They are vibrant, beautiful souls with talents, gifts, hopes and dreams, just like yours. Diseases from unsafe water and lack of basic sanitation kill more people every year than all forms of violence, including war. One billion people live without water. (12)

- Be part of World Water Day: http://www.waterday.org/.

- Here are some interesting global stats on water that will shock you:http://pacinst.org/pu.../10-shocking-facts-about-worlds-water/.

Finally, may your thirst be met with the waters of vitality throughout your travels! Cheers to optimal hydration on every journey! Yes, proper hydration will keep you out of trouble. Do keep in mind that dehydration is one of the most common reasons why any traveler lands in the emergency room.

Chapter 5

Sleep: Absolutely Essential for Vibrant Health

*Now I see the secret of making the best person: it is to grow in
the open air and to eat and sleep with the earth.*
~ Walt Whitman

In *Macbeth*, Shakespeare called sleep "the chief nourisher of life's feast." I completely agree and would add that nothing impacts our sustainable health, good moods and a "get-up-and-go attitude" like a good night's sleep.

Whether you are taking a red-eye flight, a night train, a long bus trip or an extended car ride, one of the first things to do is a get a good night's rest the night before you leave. With most travel, you are lucky to get the seven to nine hours of rest recommended by the National Sleep Foundation, let alone even a two-hour cycle without interruptions.

Lack of quality sleep is, perhaps, one of the most common travel-related concerns from which most people suffer. We often disregard our body clocks, and at a price. Moderate- and long-term sleep deprivation can lead to attention deficit disorder, weight gain and increased insulin and cortisol levels. You may already know that cortisol is a stress hormone involved in many disorders. As explained in Chapter 3, an increased cortisol level can generate sugar dysregulation, irritability, heart palpitations, anxiety, weight gain, depression and problems with learning and memory. Sustained high cortisol levels cause adrenal fatigue, which can be a contributing factor in conditions such as fibromyalgia, hypothyroidism, chronic fatigue and arthritis.

With more than 70 different types of sleep disorders that result in reduced sleep quantity or quality, it is not surprising to hear Dr. Dave Woynarowski state, "Sleep problems are one of the most common, dangerous and sadly overlooked health hazards." Some of these hazards include obstructive sleep apnea, narcolepsy, chronic insomnia, periodic limb movement disorders and circadian rhythm disorders.(1)

As a Doctor of Chinese medicine, I warn my patients that when you mess with your circadian rhythms, or your body's clock, you mess with your hormones, your digestive system, and for that matter, all of the body's organ systems. Your circadian rhythms regulate your chemical and hormonal production and metabolism along an approximate 24-hour cycle. With erratic travel schedules, many people experience brain fog, increased anxiety, belly bloat, swollen ankles and constipation.

One thing to know is that our bodies are brilliant at keeping us healthy, and our organ systems strive for homeostasis more than anything. If we find ourselves chronically stressed out, eating offensive food and overdoing it without adequate rest, at some point our body will start to break down. This does not have to happen to the HCT who follows The 8 Pathways in this book.

Are you among the fortunate people who regularly wake up refreshed, energized and ready to take on a new day after a night of restful, uninterrupted sleep? Or are you among the growing population of people who once slept well and now struggle most nights to get the deep, restorative rest that your body craves after busy, fully scheduled days and weeks? It is a rare day in my practice that I don't hear at least a few of my patients, colleagues or support staff complain of sleep deprivation. This is especially true for my patients who travel frequently.

Answer the following questions:

• Do you wake up between 1 and 3 a.m. nightly?

• Do you toss and turn all night long?

- Are your legs restless?
- Do you have trouble falling asleep or staying asleep?
- Do you have trouble quieting the incessant chatter of your mind?
- Do you wake up feeling exhausted, like you need to go back to bed?
- Is your mind foggy most days?
- Do you find that sleep is even more difficult with travel, hotels and with time zone changes?

If you answered yes to most of these questions, fear not, there are solutions. Also, know that you are not alone. Unfortunately, we live in a sleep-deprived world. A hundred years ago we might have slept nine or more hours each night, while presently, many of us average only six hours of sleep or less. Many of my patients have struggled with sleep issues for their entire life, which has contributed to lost income, stress, poor performance and even failed relationships.

Children and Sleep Disorders

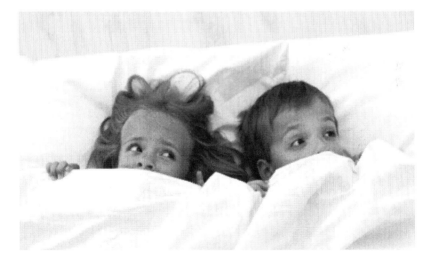

These days, more and more children are challenged with sleep issues, and it is not fun to travel when your kids don't sleep well.

As I mentioned in the Introduction, while participating in "Career Day" at my children's elementary school, I spoke to two groups of children about my practice as a Doctor of Oriental Medicine. I asked both groups if they had any trouble sleeping. At least half of the kids in each group raised their hands! Sleep deprivation is one of the negative consequences of Wi-Fi in schools, according to Magda Havas Ph.D., an expert on the hazards of Wi-Fi and increased electromagnetic exposure for children in our computerized, screened world. Children are on cell phones as early as five years of age and teenagers are often plugged in 24/7 to their Wi-Fi and iPods. Sadly, young people are spending more time exposed to these frequencies and less time outdoors in the life-promoting earth frequencies.

There's a correlation between chronic loss of sleep that occurs during infancy and early childhood and childhood obesity that can show up as early as the age of seven. In a press release on May 19, 2014, Dr. Elsie Taveras, chief of General Pediatrics at Massachusetts General Hospital for Children and lead author of the study, stated, "Our study found convincing evidence that getting less than recommended amounts of sleep across early childhood is an independent and strong risk factor for obesity."

Dr. Taveras made the following recommendations for better sleep patterns for children:(2)

1. **Set a consistent bedtime**
2. **Limit caffeinated beverages and high-sugar foods late in the day**
3. **Cut out high-tech and bright light distractions in a child's bedroom**

I will add: never use a baby monitor within 3 feet of your baby's head, and do not have the handheld device in your bedroom near your head. Most of these units emit high EMF frequencies and can cause sleepless nights and are not healthy for a growing brain.

Statistics on Sleep

The National Highway Traffic Safety Administration conservatively estimates that 100,000 police-reported crashes are the direct result of driver fatigue each year and half of those accidents involve drivers between the ages of 16 to 25.(3)

According to the findings of an expert panel published in *Sleep Health: The Journal of the National Sleep Foundation,* teenagers between the ages of 14 and 17 require 8 to 10 hours of sleep each night. The study has also found that a one-hour difference in the amount of sleep that teenagers get can greatly affect the results of their driving habits and likeliness to be involved in an auto accident. These teens are included in the estimated 1,550 deaths, 71,000 injuries, and $12.5 billion in monetary losses each year, which may just be the tip of the iceberg, since it is difficult to solidly correlate crashes to sleep deprivation while driving.(4)

The Institute of Medicine of the National Academies' Committee on Sleep Medicine and Research reports that 50 to 70 million Americans are regularly deprived of sleep or suffer from sleep disturbances. This means that up to one-sixth of the American population is affected by this disorder. The resulting daily fatigue may be good for Starbuck's bottom line and for Big Pharma, who supply sleep medications to the millions, but it's not good for your body, brain and definitely not good if you're interested in longevity.

More disconcerting sleep statistics:(4)

- 40 million people in the U.S. have a chronic sleep disorder

- The average person wakes up six times per night

- An estimated 10 million Americans and millions worldwide have undiagnosed sleep disorders

- The estimated cost to US employers is $18 billion in lost productivity due to sleep-loss issues

Sleep time is when your body repairs and your nervous system gets a break from the challenges and stress of the day. It's during sleep that you reset your body for the next day. It's a time for every system in your body to recalibrate and rejuvenate to give you optimum energy and clarity for each new moment. Sleep also helps reduce inflammation in your body and thereby helps you age more beautifully.

Extreme sleep deprivation can lead to psychosis, as demonstrated in military recruits, night-shift workers and some medical students. People who pull all-nighters on a regular basis should know that sleep deprivation spikes the levels of the hormone

ghrelin, known to be one of the "hunger hormones," which is released primarily in the stomach and thought to send signals to the
brain that then increases your appetite. It also lowers the appetite-
suppressing hormone known as peptide YY (PYY), which is a peptide secreted by cells in the lower part of the small intestine. This
hormone causes a sense of satiety, that is to say, it makes you feel
satisfied and curbs your hunger. You then tend to eat more to compensate for lack of sleep and you crave more sugars and refined
carbohydrates. As a result, sleep deprivation tends to make you
gain weight, which can lead to diabetes, heart disease and other
chronic diseases.

It gets even worse for women. Sleep deprivation is also found
to impact how estrogen is broken down in the body, often leading
to a growth in mutagenic cells and an increase in estrone. Estrone
is a type of estrogen commonly found in estrogen-dominant cancers, including breast and uterine cancers. In this case, hormones
that can cause cell mutation dramatically increase when you have
an abnormal sleep cycle.

Another factor to consider are the little "bugs" we are more
susceptible to when we travel, including bacteria, virus, fungus and
parasites. As an HCT, you want to continually be aware of your gut
ecology and to be sure that you have enough reserve of the prebiotics and probiotics, or healthy bacteria. Trust me, you do not want
to become a happy home to these microbes. (See the discussion in
Chapter 2.) It is known that parasites, in particular, come alive at
night and can also keep you awake and cause your cortisol levels
to remain high. Additionally, sleep deprivation causes stress, which
leads to more restless nights, which further degrades your health.

Pilots, Flight Attendants and Sleep Deprivation

There has been real concern about pilots who are fatigued. After
the crash of Colgan Air Flight 3407 in upstate New York on February
12, 2009, the FAA determined that the pilot's abilities had been affected by fatigue. Shortly after the crash, the FAA set a minimum
10-hour rest period prior to flight duty. A while ago, I met a pilot
who works for Fedex, who said he travels through 7 time zones in 1

week! Sleep continues to be an issue for him, and he feel strongly that his regular exercise program and hydration habits allow him to keep this rigorous lifestyle.

Little attention has been paid to the health of flight attendants. Flight attendants often work long hours with little rest, and they are human and can make critical mistakes. Improperly stowed baggage, forgetting to engage or disarm emergency chutes or neglecting other safety duties can occur as a result of long hours and little rest. "They're showing up to work impaired," stated Peter Roma, a researcher for the Federal Aviation Administration (FAA) who helped to conduct studies on sleep deprivation affecting flight attendants. The FAA considers them to be "safety professionals" so it is especially important that they are alert and can function well, if necessary, in an emergency.(5)

I talk to flight attendants all the time, and especially in preparation for this book. They have a big and demanding job and have expressed every travel complaint that has been covered in this book. They love to travel yet know their job comes with a lot of challenges. Long hours, poor food options, lifting heavy luggage, dealing with cranky travelers and exposure to radiation and other chemicals are among the most common. If you are a flight attendant or pilot that cares about your health, I am sure you have already been enlightened by what has been discussed in the previous chapters. Continue reading, as I have some more good stuff to share with you!

44-Year-Old Woman Recovers from a 25-Year Sleep Problem

For 25 years, starting in high school until 2008, I battled a serious sleeping problem. While in college, I was desperate to try anything, so I started doing yoga. I also did the complete training in Transcendental Meditation (TM) and would sit in my freshman dorm room for 20 minutes, 2 times a day, chant my mantra and sail away. Unfortunately, there was no immediate change in my sleep patterns. I also tried to be less addicted to the sugar-laden food and caffeinated drinks provided in the dining halls. Yes, I must admit, I did thrive on the consciousness shift that was happening to me through my meditation practice in 1983, yet I still remained sleepless.

My struggle continued, even with exercise, meditation and mostly good eating habits that I practiced at that time. No matter how desperate I was, I just would not give in and take a prescription drug. I went to student health many times for this condition but received little constructive counsel. I even took a stress management course designed for senior students worrying about their future. I was the only first-year student in the class, and I was grateful to pick up many useful tools that I still use today in my practice.

I learned then, in 1983, which certainly holds true today, that stress is at the root cause of many diseases and certainly is the cause of many sleep disorders. My teacher felt I was a Type A personality and that I needed to re-assess my expectations of myself. She also told me that I was fortunate to be doing all the right things health wise but that my excessive marathon running training might be a factor in my sleeplessness. She added that I needed to learn to ride the good stress (eustress) wave, in order not to break down and get sick.

I tried all kinds of herbs and sleep-elixir teas, and when I went to acupuncture school, I would brew just about every stress-release and sleep-enhancing, terrible-tasting concoction you could imagine. Each formula had eight or ten different barks, flowers and even bones, all known to help one sleep. I did blood tests and hormone tests to get to the root of my problem. Not one thing was clearly shown to be the source of my sleep disturbance, and although a remedy might help for a day or two, nothing seemed to help long-term.

Seemingly helpless, I found myself on the treatment tables of shamans, medical doctors, nurse practitioners, intuitive counselors and energy healers. I spent a lot of time in tears, feeling alone and pretty crazy some days just from the sleep deprivation. I would have a few months where the condition would subside, and then again, it would be followed by a few more rough months.

As time went on, I managed to build my practice, and it was thriving. I married and gave birth to two children, and continued to travel the world to learn about the best health practices, including herbalism, acupuncture, touch therapy and shamanic therapies, with the goal in mind to solve the world's growing health problems, including insomnia.

After consulting with my friends and local colleagues Paula Baker-Laporte and Erica Elliott, M.D., authors of *Prescriptions for a Healthy House,* I began wondering if my home could be the root cause of my sleep issues.

In 2008, I finally solved my sleep issues. I hired Dan Stih, author of *Healthy Living Spaces.* I thought perhaps my house was infested with mold and was the probable culprit impacting my sleep and sinuses. What I found to be the truth astounded me. Dan told me that the biggest health hazard in my home were the high intensity frequencies that were coming from a water tower above our house (that supplies water to 10,000 people), which had at least 15 telecommunication devices on top of it. He used a $4,000 gauss meter, which revealed that the intensity of the frequencies emanating from the tower were much higher than the meter could even measure. Check out this photo:

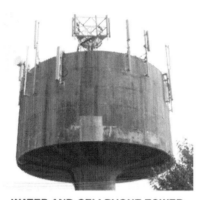

WATER AND CELLPHONE TOWER

Water tower above my house, surrounded by 15 to 20 telecommunication devices.

A few weeks later, I was introduced to an earthing technology called pulsed electromagnetic field (PEMF) by John Gray, author of *Men Are from Mars, Women Are from Venus,* when he spoke for my nonprofit event. In fact, Dr. Gray shared his enthusiasm for this FDA-registered wellness device to a sold out audience in Santa Fe, NM. He believes this PEMF device to be one of the best technologies he has come across in his 30-year career in the health and fitness world, and he encouraged me to use this in my health center.

The device is a magnetic resonance machine that delivers its natural frequencies (like the earth naturally provides) by way of a mat that you lay out on a massage table, on your bed, or on the floor. The mat has six copper Tesla coils inside it that creates frequencies to restore your body to the low frequencies (Green Zone, see Figure A, in the Introduction) of the earth after only an eight-minute session.

After using the PEMF mat for several days, I began to sleep deeply, in a way I had not known for most of my life. I discovered that my body was in the Yellow/Red Zone and that my nervous system was completely unbalanced. I was driving too much of my sympathetic nervous system (the yang, get-up-and-go system) by living in a home that was highly toxic due to the high levels of EMF pollution coming from all the telecommunications above my home, and for years sleeping with a clock radio near my head.

Other contributing factors to my sleeplessness were marathon running, overworking and not getting adequate rest. All of this kept my body in the alarm Red Zone, which is the way many people live in today's world (and often with a chronic disease). Therefore, the parasympathetic part of my nervous system (the yin, digest, rest and repair cycle) was not being supported. The mat technology was supplying me with the low level yin frequencies that helped restore my failing parasympathetic nervous system due to my lifestyle choices. Once I discovered and understood the mechanism of this PEMF technology and continued using it, I was finally able to enjoy deep sleep and restore my body from years of being in the Red Zone (see Chapter 1, Electrified Times Chart) and learn more in Chapter 7).

I am excited to report that I have helped hundreds of people restore their sleep issues by solving my own sleep nightmare and following suggestions and sleep solutions I offer in this chapter.

Little did I know that this finding would forever change the course of my life, my practice and why I had to write this book. It changed my life because I could finally sleep and get my sanity back. It changed my practice because I made it a standard routine to help each of my patients understand the value of upgrading the electrical nature of their bodies by creating beautiful, healthy cells (grape cells instead of dried-out, raisin-looking cells as discussed in Chapter 1). Your body and your cells are like a battery. When you are well and thriving, your battery is charged (Green Zone). When you are sick and are suffering from a chronic disease, your battery (voltage) is low (Yellow and Red Zone).

The best way to keep your body fully charged is to be outdoors as often as possible (and when you are unable to use a PEMF mat or earthing device that mimics nature, or other forms of energy medicine like acupuncture and Reiki), drink clean water with minerals, eat a plant-rich diet, and avoid the artificial frequencies of modern life when possible and to not let stress eat you up from the inside out. As Walt Whitman says, "Now I know the secrets of a making the best person; it is to grow in the open air and to eat and sleep from the earth."

Traveling often is the perfect storm where we challenge our core electrical nature by making choices that cause our body batteries to get run-down. Therefore I was inspired to write this book to help you become an HCT who follows these simple pathways to experience healthy, smart and effortless travel with each trip. Each chapter is dedicated to help you restore your body, mind and spirit and to learn how to sustain optimal health as you *travel* through life each day of your life.

The Importance of REM Sleep for the HCT

Rapid Eye Movement (REM) sleep is part of regeneration during sleep and it is very important. Overall, REM sleep is essential for processing emotions, stress and memories. Most dreaming happens during REM sleep, but it can also happen during other stages of sleep. Several different stages during sleep and REM sleep can occur in as many as six cycles in an eight-hour sleep period. This accounts for approximately two hours of the total sleep cycle. REM sleep is marked by some interesting physical activities, from the quickening of the heartbeat and eyes moving rapidly from side to side to lower body temperature and other physiologic events. During REM sleep, the muscles become paralyzed as a defense mechanism. This actually keeps us from hurting ourselves while acting out some of the contents of our dreams. You might have noticed that sometimes, when waking up from a sound sleep, your mind can be awake but you cannot move for a bit due to this temporary state of paralysis. If you are unaware of the reason, it can be pretty scary.

Additionally, better REM sleep helps to support your good moods during the day, so it would be especially helpful to get REM sleep as much as possible while traveling. You will learn about REM sleep-boosting strategies as you continue reading. The REM sleep stage is longer in the morning, so try to sleep a bit longer in the morning. Try this and see if you notice that your mood improves.(6)

Getting proper sleep

According to Ayurvedic and Chinese medicine, the ideal hours for sleep are between 9:00 p.m. and 6:00 a.m. By staying awake when you should ideally be sleeping, or vice versa, can work against your biology, interfere with your hormones and cause fluctuations of melatonin, serotonin, cortisol and insulin growth factor (IGF). As we consider the merits of regular, sustained nights of deep rest, it is easy to see how all forms of travel can thwart this most important pathway to achieving optimal health.

I recommend to all my patients when traveling by car and experiencing sleeplessness, to immediately pull over to a safe area along the road. What I do when this happens is to get out of my car and do several jumping jacks or carefully run around the car. Or you could try rolling down the window and letting in some cool fresh air. Scream, slap awake your 22 facial muscles (I just love anatomy!) or make a call to a loved one. It is best not to get in this situation in the first place, but just in case, know what to do!

Instead of engaging in a Red Bull caffeine habit, incorporate a healthy lifestyle that provides adequate rest and supports your energy needs. Caffeine does have a place now and then, but rather than trying to boost your tired body with supplements, let me share with you some tried-and-true healthier ways.

10 ACTION STEPS TO ENSURE DEEP, RESTORATIVE SLEEP AND REST DURING TRAVEL

1. **Go to bed and wake up the same time, as often as possible**. This is recommended throughout life and is considered to be the foundation in Chinese medicine. Even when traveling, try to stay on your regular sleep cycle when you can. It is easy to see how much your body prefers 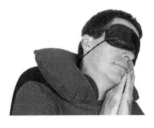 a regular sleep schedule when it's time to turn our clock forward or back one hour, twice a year. The end of Daylight Savings Time

does exacerbate sleep difficulties, depression and, year after year, is a time when there are more sleep-related accidents.

Our bodies are cyclical, and have a propensity for what is regular and routine. Our bodies are designed to be well and will do what is possible to keep the balance, also known as homeostasis. When you throw your body off track with irregular sleep patterns, it can wreak havoc with everything from your moods to productivity. Follow the recommendations here and always do your best to get back on track.

2. **Alcohol and deep restorative rest do not go together**. If sleep problems are an issue for you, avoid alcohol altogether. Alcohol sugar completely throws off your blood sugar and is one of the main reasons people feel their heart racing while trying to sleep. Like anything, some people are more sensitive than others. If you're serious about getting restorative sleep, avoid alcohol, at least a few hours before bed.

3. **Electro-sanitize your room**. (See Chapters 8 and 10.) Check your bedroom and/or hotel room or any room you stay in while traveling for negative electromagnetic fields (EMFs). To do this, you need a gauss meter. You can find various models online for $150 to $450. Some experts even recommend at home pulling your circuit breaker before bed, to shut down all the power in your house. At least, turn off your bedroom Wi-Fi router!

Recent studies have linked electromagnetic frequencies (EMFs), a type of low-frequency radiation emitted from your computer, television set, microwave, mobile phone and cordless phone, with an increase in lymphoma, brain cancer, melanoma, breast cancer, leukemia, miscarriage, birth defects, suicide and even Alzheimer's disease. EMFs are also known to disrupt your pineal gland and lower the production of melatonin. Ouch, this is not good for quality sleep!

Recently, Malka N. Halgamuge of the University of Melbourne in Australia, studied the effect of man-made EMFs on the pineal gland. Given the evidence of his research, Halgamuge believes that it is likely that the pineal gland recognizes these frequencies as light. It follows that melatonin production would be reduced. He states in the *Oxford Journal*, "The results show the significance of disruption of melatonin due to exposure to weak EMFs, which may possibly lead to long-term health effects in humans." EMFs are also known to depress a brain chemical called serotonin. The reduction of both melatonin and serotonin is associated with mood changes, depression and psychiatric disorders.(7)

Unplug everything around your head. Move alarm clocks and other electrical devices away from your bed. If these devices must be used, keep them as far away from your bed as possible, but at least six feet from you. Turn off all computers, iPods, cell phones and Kindle devices at least two hours before bed in order to create some distance from these stimulating yet exhausting frequencies. Yes, even Kindles, Nooks and iPads put out electromagnetic fields and light that can keep you in a hyper-alert state.

4. One of the best ways to stimulate melatonin production naturally in your body is to **sleep in a completely dark room**. If this is not possible, due to moonlight or outdoor lights that cannot be turned off outside your bedroom, try to get in the habit of wearing a sleep mask that completely blocks out all light. This will also come in handy for sleep time on a plane as well. (See below for more information.) Melatonin is a very important hormone that is produced in your body and is very important for normal sleep cycles. Melatonin has been shown in many clinical studies around the world to inhibit cancer cell growth. Low levels of melatonin have also been shown to *stimulate* cancer cell growth.

Did you know that a handful of raw walnuts has been demonstrated to triple your blood levels of melatonin, not to mention walnuts give you healthy omega-3s? If you must eat something before you sleep, raw organic walnuts it is.

Remember, nighttime is when you want minimal exposure to all light. Even small amounts of light at night suppress melatonin release and skew our circadian clock, making good sleep difficult and promoting weight gain.

Ann Louise Gittleman asks, "But how exactly does this lack of sleep cause weight gain? Sleeping less than at least seven or eight hours a night inhibits the body's ability to metabolize carbohydrates, leading to higher insulin levels and eventually, Type 2 diabetes. And it also contributes to the nationwide obesity epidemic–people who slept only five hours a night have been found 74% more likely to become obese than those who slept for seven to nine hours nightly, according to data from the National Health and Nutrition Examination Study."(8)

5. If at all possible, **keep your window open a bit**, even in the winter, to allow fresh air into the room. I am always thrilled to stay in hotel rooms where the windows are open. I sleep much better and welcome air from the outdoors. Indoor air is often dry, recycled and full of unknown contaminants. To keep it simple, there is everything from dust particles to mold, rug and furniture chemicals that outgas formaldehydes and other offensive substances.

If there is noise that disturbs you, use a white noise machine, a meditation app or turn on the radio to a soft, classical-music station. I use a sound machine almost every night of my life, as I am a light sleeper. Fortunately most of my travel roommates are amenable to this habit of mine. I consider it part of my healthy travel blueprint. You will learn more about creating your healthy travel blueprint in Chapter 8. (See # 8 below.)

6. **Finish your last meal or snack three hours before bed**, so your body is not spending sleep time digesting when this is your time to repair on a cellular level (REM sleep).Listen to your inner self (Pathway 8) that knows it is best not to eat sugar or drink caffeinated or alcoholic beverages before sleep.

7. **Take a warm bath before bedtime** with relaxing aromatherapy essential oils or add some bath salts to relieve the aches and pains of your day. You could stretch or do some yoga poses and sip calming teas, like chamomile, just before bed.

8. **Listen to soothing music to relax**. There are unlimited choices online, including subliminal meditation, hypnosis for sleep, and a myriad of other sleep technologies. Also consider lying on a pulsed electromagnetic frequency (PEMF) mat.(See Chapter 10.) These mats often include a sound and light machine that helps to engage the theta and delta brain waves that are needed for sleep. (See Chapter 6.)

9. **Write your gratitude statements for the day** *each* night before bed. This practice has been found to help people release the stress of the day by focusing on what was satisfying and heart-nurturing, even on hectic and difficult days. You can find your gratitude journal at amazon.com. Also consider keeping a dream journal and record your nightly dreams while you travel. You'll be amazed at what you can interpret from your nocturnal reveries, and writing things down before you go to sleep can help trigger what you dream about and where your dreams take you.

10. If your sleep issues are severe and all the above steps are not helping, **consider getting an evaluation from a clinic specializing in sleep disorders**. Also, hypnotherapy, acupuncture, regular massage and other modalities can help to remedy your sleep problems. Also, listen to a great interview with sleep expert Dr. Michael Breus (Dr. Oz's sleep doctor) at <u>www.healthytravelers summit.com</u>.

Dr. Benson's fast-track sleep cure for travel

S-L-E-E-P:

S-hut all light out of your room and/or wear a comfortable sleep mask.

L-et go of the day, be in the moment and breathe, meditate or write in your travel journal.

E-lectro-sanitize your sleeping space by unplugging all electronics at least two hours before bed. Remember to charge your phone in any other room but your bedroom.

E-arthing before bed, walk barefoot on the grass or at the beach on the sand. Take in Mother Earth's frequencies, or use a PEMF device, earthing sheet or mat.

P-lan for your next day a few hours before you sleep. That could involve planning your food for the day, your exercise plan, sights to see and work to complete, so that you are not figuring this out in the middle of the night while trying to sleep.

Six steps to overcome jet lag

Jet lag is no fun! Lets face it, no one feels good after traveling through several time zones. As an avid international traveler, I know this feeling intimately, and I have tried everything I have researched to help reduce the effects of jet lag. I recommend that you review the Healthy Conscious 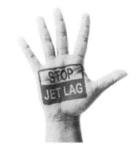 Traveler's Blueprint as outlined in Chapter 8, to allow your body to experience smoother travel zone transitions.

Truth be told, jet lag has kicked my butt, even knowing how best to prevent a serious case of it. One time when I traveled to

Switzerland, I went to a Cheap Trick concert the evening that I arrived. I slept through 95% of the concert and you would not believe how loud it was (what I did remember). I missed most of *The Lion King* on Broadway and other great shows when I traveled only two time zones away. I even slept through a performance by a renowned New York comedian. Maybe it was because he really was not that funny. But what I was really bummed out about most was when I slept through a full three-hour bus tour of London during my first visit. I did manage to get out and shop at Harrods, but that was all I remember. After all I have researched for this chapter, I feel much more confident to get this down to a better science, so I don't miss out anymore on life's great pleasures and sights.

1. Get an **acupuncture** or massage reset treatment when possible, to help your body get attuned to the new time zone. Acupuncture is a great choice to calm your nervous system after erratic sleep patterns. It also reduces inflammation, helps your body detox harmful substances and balances your hormones.

2. Maintain your **hydration** schedule in order to avoid jet lag and also to recover more quickly from international travel.

3. Consume the HCT anti-inflammatory **good food** program outlined in Chapter 2. These foods are unprocessed, low in sodium and nutrient rich. Also, international travel is the perfect time to eat less, especially when you are not moving much in tight airplane seats. I also recommend Dr. Charles Ehret's *Anti-Jet Lag Diet*. He has extensively researched human circadian rhythms and the effect diet has on jet lag. His research reveals that those who use his diet are seven times less likely to experience jet lag when traveling eastward and sixteen times less likely when traveling westward. You can look at his website, which allows you to enter in your personal details and create an individualized plan for yourself. You can find this at: www.stopjetlag.com, and the basics of the diet are also available online at www.netlib.org/misc/jet-lag-diet.

4. Supplement the sleep hormone **melatonin** before your newly desired sleep time, at least a few days in advance. This helps reduce jet lag. It is best to support your own production of melatonin by blocking out as much light as possible when you sleep each night. It is worth repeating: when there is light entering your room at night, it prevents your pineal gland from naturally producing melatonin. It is helpful to supplement with .3- 3 mg of melatonin before,

during and after international travel. Just find a brand that you like. Once you have taken melatonin for one to two weeks, get off of it and allow your own body to make its own melatonin. You can also take it when you go through periodic times of sleeplessness to get back on track.

5. Try bright **light therapy**. Strong light entering our eyes helps to reset your circadian rhythm. Some people bring portable medical lamps on trips, however an easier way of doing this is to get up at the new desired waking time, such as 7:00 a.m., and immediately sit outside with direct sun hitting your face for 10 minutes. And when you arrive to your new destination early in the morning, continue to be out in the bright, natural light and avoid taking a siesta that might endure your jet lag.

6. Research has shown that **earthing**, i.e., being electrically connected to the earth, helps reset circadian rhythms. When we fly high above the earth, we are in an ungrounded state. The simplest way to ground ourselves is to spend 15 to 20 minutes outdoors with the soles of your feet touching the earth in your new location.(9)

Essential sleep products

1. **Eye covers**: Tempurpedic is my favorite brand because it is very comfortable and it blocks out all light. I do recommend letting it air out, outside the box for a few days before you use it if there is any outgassing. Cover your eyes at night to increase melatonin production and REM sleep. Year after year, maintaining adequate levels of melatonin by covering your eyes will be a great practice for aging well. Any light, especially flickering lights of cell phones and computers, can severely impact your body's ability to go into a deep REM sleep and are known to increase restless sleep.

2. **Earthing sheets and pads**: The combination of natural cotton and silver threads in a sheet or pad can provide you with a tool for grounding and lead to deeper, more regenerative sleep. (See Chapter 10.)

3. **Herbal sleep teas**, such as chamomile, passionflower, hops, catnip and lemon balm, can help to remedy sleeplessness. You can find blends of these herbs in organic commercial teas.

4. **Essential oils**, such as lavender (sprayed on your pillow), is highly recommended. Other choices include clary sage, frankincense,

marjoram, orange, rosemary, ylang ylang or blends like Peace and Calming or Surrender from Young Living Oils (http://www.young living.com/en_US) or Serenity and Balance from Doterra (http://www.doterra.com/#/en). These have very good relaxing or sedative properties.

5. **Sound machines** are available in an array of choices, offering natural sounds as well as white noise. It's best to try out a few before purchasing, since certain sounds can be annoying to some people. I am a light sleeper, so I never leave home without mine!

6. For anyone with **snoring issues**, or the partner or friend of someone who snores, check out SnoreWorld.com, devoted to helping the world get a good night's sleep. Nose strips can work for some people who snore, and these can be found at most drugstores.

As it turns out, eighteen million people in the U.S. suffer from sleep apnea. If this is at the core of your problem, it's important to be assessed by a health professional specializing in this area. The best sleep travel apnea machine I have discovered can be found in Chapter 10.

Natural sleep supplements

According to the U.S. Food and Drug Administration (FDA) data, over-the-counter (OTC) sleep products, such as Excedrin PM and Tylenol PM, don't offer any significant benefit to patients. In 2007, an analysis of studies on various prescriptive sleeping aids, financed by the National Institutes of Health (NIH), found that sleeping pills like Ambien, Lunesta and Sonata reduced the average time to go to sleep by just under 13 minutes, compared to sugar pills. That's hardly a major improvement! HCT, my advice is to find natural ways to get a good night's rest. Here are my favorite suggestions, but most importantly, remember to follow The 8 Pathways to get a good night's rest, every night.

Magnesium is a great multi-purpose mineral that is integral to at least 200 biological processes, including healthy heart function and optimal bone formation and integrity. It also has anti-spasmodic properties. Magnesium is known for its calming nature and for promoting healthy bowel movements. 300-600 mg of chelated magnesium at night is recommended. A popular brand is called CALM by Natural Vitality.

An Mien Pien is a popular Chinese medicine formula that calms the heart and mind and helps to restore a healthy nervous system. Traditional Chinese medicine teaches us that the heart is considered the "seat of the spirit." It follows that if the yin, or nourishing aspect of the heart, is depleted, this will result in anxiety, restlessness and insomnia.

Tryptophan is a potent amino acid that not only elevates mood by increasing serotonin levels, but also helps to reduce anxiety. A 500 mg dose can often be helpful for the occasional bout of insomnia.

Melatonin helps to regulate sleep patterns. Melatonin levels decrease with age, which is why it's important to supplement this loss for better sleep patterns. Start with .3 - 1 mg and work up to 3 mg, if needed. Alter your intake with international travel, or consider only taking for jet lag, depending on your sleep needs and concerns. According to Dr. Christine Horner:

Melatonin is not only our sleep hormone, but it also is a very powerful antioxidant. It decreases the amount of estrogen our body produces. It also boosts your immune system. . . And it interacts with the other hormones. So, if you go to bed after 10:00 p.m., [the later hour] significantly increases your risk of breast cancer.(10)

L-Theanine is an amino acid derived from herbal teas. Commonly found in green tea, it can calm your mind. This amino acid is thought to have a relaxing effect on the mind by increasing alpha-wave activity. Relaxation is an essential part of falling asleep.

Gaba is an amino acid sometimes known as natural Valium. The growing world population is becoming increasingly deficient in this substance as more people present with anxiety, sleeplessness, irritability and restlessness due to all the reasons outlined in this book. I find this to be exceptionally useful for sound sleep. However, I often prescribe it to my patients to take it first thing in the morning to help ensure a calm day no matter what the circumstances are. I too will take Gaba during stressful days at the office, and I find that my mind stays calm and sharp, rather than going into overwhelm.

Phenitropic from Biotics Research Corporation contains a derivative of Gaba and has been shown to have a calming effect, which can improve impaired sleep. This is one of the most popular sleep remedies I use at my clinic.

Valerian Extract is a perennial herb that has been used for centuries to promote relaxation and sleep. Valerian is thought to help improve the amount of time it takes to fall asleep and the quality of sleep. Some people do not do well with Valerian and too much of it can be toxic for your liver. Several patients of mine love it.

Lemon Balm is also a perennial herb in the mint family that has been used for centuries to promote relaxation and sleep. It is credited with promoting a calm and relaxed state of mind, which is an important part of falling asleep.

Hops Extract, which is from the female flowers of the hops plant, in combination with valerian can help increase alpha-waves. This then helps to reduce the amount of time it takes to fall asleep and also improves the quality of sleep. The popular folk remedy for sleeplessness is a "pillow filled with hops."

Passion Flower is a truly beautiful flower that is also well known for its calming effects, apart from its vibrant colors and unique appearance. Passion flower is traditionally used to promote sleep, and you can drink it as a tea.

Chamomile Flower is a daisy-like flower that is well known for its calming effects and use in herbal teas. It is traditionally used to promote calmness and sleep.

Cherries are one of the few known food sources of melatonin. Tart montmorency cherries are loaded with the potent antioxidant melatonin, produced naturally by the body's pineal gland. Try taking a tablespoon in four ounces of water before bedtime.

Call to action:

- If you have a sleep issue, make it your #1 priority to get it resolved and consider many of the suggestions in this chapter.

- Invest in an earthing device or PEMF device to bring the power of nature's frequencies into your home, 24/7, to help balance your nervous system.

- Seriously look at your schedule, your home and people clutter, and let go of anything that is not absolutely necessary in your life. You need the digest, rest and restore part of your body working as much as you need the go button on, to be a HCT throughout life.
- Memorize the S.L.E.E.P acronym.

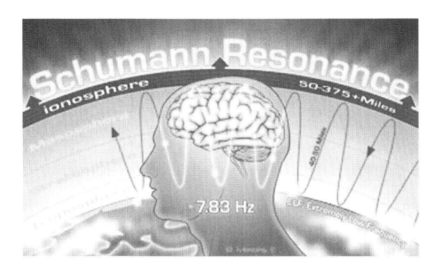

Chapter 6

Travel with Optimal Moods, Brain Power and Stress Resiliency

*To live a life of virtue, match up your thoughts, words and
deeds. ~ Epictetus*

People today spend an enormous amount of their lives traveling by artificial means. It is not natural to cross three time zones by plane, travel in a car, or spend the day on a motorcycle or train. These modern-day travel choices stress the body, drain the brain, and create foul moods! In this chapter you will discover how to reset your travel with more pleasant moods, minimal stress and a smart brain.

Would you travel more if there was a guarantee that travel could be stress-free, that your brain would stay sharp and you could sustain pleasant moods? Though these experiences are currently rare for the frequent traveler, this chapter will teach you how travel can actually be more fun.

I interviewed more than 100 flight attendants, 30 pilots, endless TSA agents, truck drivers and hundreds of travelers, including many of my patients who travel frequently. The most common complaints they listed were fatigue, sensitivity to sounds and smells, moodiness, brain fog, loss of memory, stress, sleeplessness, tight neck and shoulders, sitting too close to fellow passengers on planes, fussy children and *crappy* food choices.

I agree with Dr. Norm Shealy that the ever-increasing pace and stress of modern life can easily pull us off track and back into the conditioned and often neurotic ego mind. Travel definitely can put you in a consistent stress response if you allow it. Stress is often the root of why most people get sick, have anxiety attacks, palpitations and end up in their doctor's office. According to the American Institute of Stress (AIS), it is estimated that 75 to 90% of all visits to primary care physicians are for stress-related problems.(1)

One of the gifts of travel is to truly test your humanity, your ability to stay in your integrity, to practice loving kindness and to see just how calm, cool and collected you can stay when the common frustrations of travel challenge your core self. Because I travel frequently, I have a lot of opportunity to practice what I am sharing in this chapter. What I do know for sure is that although I cannot control unexpected delays and traffic jams, I can control how I respond and perceive these events and how quickly I *can regain* my moods, emotions, and focused thinking. The other option is to choose to have a bad day, feel like a victim and miss out on accepting what is. Obviously, I would rather be present for the opportunity that is being offered to me.

Eckhart Tolle has brilliantly stated that the ego seeks out, and attaches itself to things that are just substitutes for the being it cannot feel." Think about that. I carry this quote with me everywhere I go and it helps me to quickly course correct, and to prevent what I cannot control from consuming me. Simple conscious choices, like reframing events, can set you free from your own emotional prison (Pathway 7). The other quote that keeps my emotions in check is from Shakespeare's *Hamlet*: "[T]here is nothing either good or bad, but thinking makes it so."

Most of us want to be aware, active, capable and engaged

when we travel! The power of our brain, thoughts and perceptions affect how we feel. I have heard that we have more than 60,000 thoughts in a single day. How many of these are actually positive thoughts? Not many! How are these negative thought patterns affecting our cells, hormones, nervous system and, thus, our total health? Negative thinking not only spoils our present moments, but also our body becomes acidic, compromising our biology and chemistry.

As you learned in Chapter 1, our electrical body responds more favorably to a balanced acid/alkaline system. If you'd like to check this out for yourself, buy pH strips and test yourself several times throughout a week. Moisten a strip on your tongue (or pee on the strip) and then look at the color, based on the chart provided. If it is bright yellow you are too acidic. This great practice can tell you a lot about your body. A quick remedy is to add organic lemon juice to your water in the morning and or apple cider vinegar to neutralize the acidity in your system.

Dr. Daniel Amen, America's favorite brain doctor, tells us to fall in love with our brains to be a superhero. "Your brain is an organ of planning, judgment and every decision you make," he says. "When your brain works right, you work right."(1) Our brains are under-functioning when we are dehydrated or when we have an excess or deficiency of certain

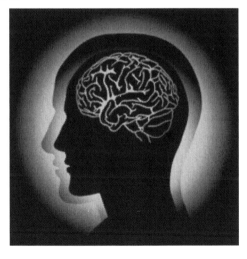

neurochemicals such as serotonin, Gaba, dopamine and norepinephrine, or minerals such as zinc, magnesium, as well as B vitamins. Phosphatide serine (PS) and acetylcarnitine are two beneficial brain nutrients that help to build and protect neurons.

Our brains also malfunction when we feed ourselves processed foods high in sugar, drink alcohol or when we spend entire days in front of the computer or TV. Just remember that your current lifestyle, moods and how you deal with stress have a major impact on the quality of your brain health.

Dr. Amen says there are four words that pertain to the essence of brain health: "*Avoid bad, do good.*"(2) I think we can agree that if we do good and follow The 8 Pathways, we will be on our way to optimal brain power.

The 8 HCT Pathways: The Real Cure for a Sharp Mind and Resilience in Spite of Stress

1. Be Your Own Best Health Care Advocate.

Live by your design and stay committed to what you innately know keeps your brain sharp, your moods elevated and your stress levels low. I treat a lot of movers and shakers who travel the world, including some who travel as much as 30 weeks each year. This lifestyle can only be maintained, without accelerated aging, by practicing the HCT 8 Pathways, and yes, number one is practicing impeccable self-care. No one can do this for you, so love and honor yourself by *doing good*!

2. Reconnect to the Earth Regularly.

It is rare to be in a bad mood when you are out in nature. Fresh, oxygenated air is medicine for a healthy brain and calms your stressed-out nervous system. The negative ions directly under your feet that come from the earth are the perfect antidote to bad moods, physical pain and depression. Connecting to the earth even increases your oxytocin, a feel-good hormone that is naturally elevated through touch, sex, and even singing or doing something new and exciting. Increasing oxytocin is great for optimizing your brain function, reducing stress and elevating your moods. *Retrain* yourself to get out more in nature when you travel, even on business trips. This way you can regain a more balanced, healthy and happy life.

In the book *Earthing*, co-author Clint Ober shares his research using electrical brain measurements from electroencephalography (EEG) and electrical skeletal muscle measurements from electromyography

(EMG) to reveal that grounding significantly influences the electrical activity of your brain and muscles. It can even take as little time as a half hour of connection to the earth. In fact, dramatic changes were recorded almost instantly within two seconds of earthing.(3)

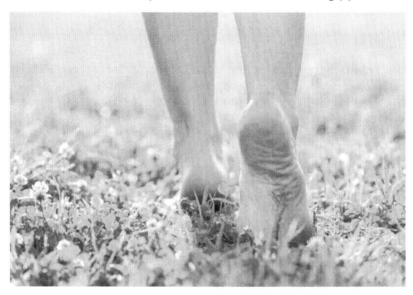

Earthing, such as walking barefoot on the earth, being connected via the grounding outlets in your home, special earthing shoes, or lying on a Tesla coil PEMF mat (Chapter 10) is the ultimate choice for anti-aging and anti-inflammation or just for simply feeling good. If you cannot get outdoors, consider investing in Ober's earthing sheets, or buy a PEMF/copper coiled mat like I have. I never travel without mine. In just eight minutes, you can use this intelligent technology that mimics the earth's frequencies to restore your under-functioning cells to healthy cells by optimizing your oxygen utilization, and removing toxins. See Chapter 10 for more information on these earthing solutions.

3. Eat Natural, Organic, GMO-free, Grass-fed, High-quality Foods.

This requires that we stay committed to our anti-inflammatory diet, which is loaded with colorful phytonutrients and carotenoids, which are plant-based nutrients and pigments that act as antioxidants. These elements are found in certain vegetables, fruits and some nuts and beans. All too often, travel can be an excuse for people to eat terribly, so it's no wonder you see a lot of moody and stressed-out people in airports, subways and on the highways.

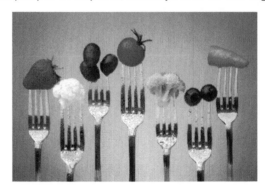

I truly believe that dehydration and poor food choices are the reason people are challenged with brain fog, lack of focus and disorientation in everyday life. This is especially evident when we fly at 30,000 feet and above, while over-consuming addictive, salty foods that are full of bad GMO oils such as canola, cottonseed and soy, not to mention hydrogenated oils that take (*wowza!*) 50 days to break down in your body! Healthy fats like DHA found in fish and eggs, omega-3s found in chia seeds, and fish and grass-fed butter are essential for a high-functioning brain. A low-fat diet is never recommended for the HCT. Our brains and our bodies thrive on healthy fats. For this reason, I pack my high-quality, low-mercury, Vital Choice canned or packaged fish on each trip. See Chapter 10 for more information.

I now also travel with Brain Octane Oil, which contains 8-carbon medium-chain triglycerides from coconut and/or palm kernel oil. It provides almost instant energy to the brain without requiring glucose from dietary sugars or carbohydrates and most importantly reduces brain fog. It's created by my friend Dave Asprey, founder and CEO of Bulletproof and author of *The New York Times* bestselling book *The Bulletproof Diet.* In addition, Brain Octane Oil gets rid of gut yeast and candida, both responsible for producing more than 180 toxic chemicals in the bloodstream. It's 18 times stronger than coconut oil for maximum cognitive function. You can listen to Asprey's (a professional biohacker) insights on travel and health at www.healthytravelerssummit.com.

Take a moment now to revisit Chapter 2 to refresh how the HCT can eat well while on the road.

4. Drink Lots of Pure Water with a Pinch of Sea Salt.

Proper hydration can ensure a trip with better moods, focus and energy and will help you adapt better to the craziness of travel. Know that even a mild case of dehydration can lead to some serious and unexpected health challenges. I learned this the hard way after traveling to Prague to run a marathon. I only gave myself 48 hours to acclimate, and after running 26 miles in the heat of the day, I landed in the hospital two hours after the marathon ended, due to a life-threatening case of dehydration and heat exhaustion. To avoid any complications of dehydration, follow the Healthy Conscious Traveler's Blueprint in Chapter 8. One severe case of dehydration can take days of life out of you and cause a seriously under-functioning brain and body. The problem is, it can creep up on you when you least expect it, so *stay* hydrated.

5. Stay Active and Exercise Your Body and Brain Daily.

This is one of the best ways to increase oxygen flow to the brain and also the flow of blood and essential nutrients to the body. Exercise removes the brain fog that often occurs during travel and car and plane trips for extended periods of time. We add *more good* to our brain and ensure good moods not just by exercising our body, but also by exercising our brain.

In terms of exercise for the brain, Jim Kwik has been my favorite expert on this topic. When I interviewed him for my www.jointheself carerevolution.com series, he said something I will never forget: "There is no such thing as good memory or bad memory—only a trained or untrained memory." Fortunately, we live in a time when there are many ways to train the brain. Your best bet is to buy one of Jim Kwik's excellent programs or books. You'll learn more about improving your mental fitness, moods and stress resiliency later in this chapter.

6. Quality Sleep Is Fundamental.

Let's face it: traveling is always a better experience when you get regular, seven to nine hours of sleep. My colleague, Dr. Glenn Wilcox, D.O.M., believes that regular sleep is essential for true good health. "This is one of the most important and overlooked factors in

American health care. There seems to be an unspoken attitude that getting enough appropriate sleep is for lazy people. What is appropriate sleep? It will vary individually, but generally a wise choice includes getting to sleep before 10:00 p.m. and sleeping deeply until you naturally wake up, without an alarm clock. For most people this will be eight to nine hours of sleep. Some people appear to function well on five or six hours, but they are certainly the exception. For comparison, the authors of *Lights Out*, a book that summarizes sleep research, explain that at the end of the 19th century, before the invention of the electric light bulb, Americans slept on average 10 hours a night. *Wow!*"

7. Be Conscious, Travel with Intention and Develop Resiliency.

Always ask yourself, how do you want to feel throughout your travels? When you have an intention or desired outcome for each trip, it is easier for your body and mind to respond. Again, this is living by design. For example, for three straight upcoming weekends, I have three different events to which I am flying—a medical conference in Dallas, a coaching event in San Diego, and a 13th birthday celebration for my daughter in New York City. Two weeks after that, I will be flying to Toronto. This might sound crazy, yet it is common in my life. I follow the HCT lifestyle and particularly follow the Healthy Conscious Traveler's Blueprint as outlined in Chapter 8. Each of these travel events are extremely important, so my intention and early preparation allows for successful, regular travel. Try having this kind of an intention and see how your travels become more productive, rewarding and full of rich memories.

8. Practice Meditation and Use Mindfulness Techniques.

There is an incredible amount of research and science that supports the efficacy of meditation and mindfulness practices, such as breathing, Tai Chi, Qi-Gong, Tapping and Yoga. I do meditate regularly and find that one of my favorite methods is a walking meditation. Thankfully, Jon Kabat Zinn wrote a fabulous book, *Full Catastrophe Living*, and qualified walking meditation as an authentic form of meditation. I am not one for sitting in lotus style. It's just not my thing. Tapping, better known as the Emotional Freedom Technique (EFT), meditation, breath work and other methods are outlined in Chapter 9. Although I am not a regular tapper, I do find it useful in stressful situations. Meditation, for sure, is one of your best choices for mental fitness. Not only is it relaxing, it teaches your mind to focus and allows you to be more resilient with the unexpected, during travel and in daily life.

This year I brought HeartMath into my daily practice and travels. I find doing 30-minute Heart Math sessions useful on planes and trains and when I am a passenger in a car. Within minutes, as I focus on my breathing and pleasant places, my nervous system relaxes, my brain sharpens and I simply feel better. This is measured by Heart Rate Variability. I have the Inner Balance App from HeartMath on my iPhone (see Chapter 10). To explain it simply, if I am seeing green on the inner balance app, I am achieving more resonance in my heart, which means my brain is also benefiting with increased focus, as there is reduced stress throughout my body.

If my brain is rapid-firing and I am stressed, more than likely I have activated ultra beta waves in my brain, which is in the Red Zone (Figure 6A). With a regular mindfulness practice and HeartMath practice, you can help retrain your brain to live more frequently in the alpha and theta zones (Green Zone). This equates to deeper sleep, more peace and happiness and fun-filled travels, no matter what happens.

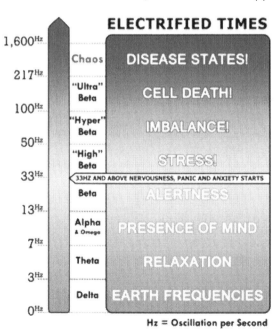

Figure 6A

This is an exciting time, not only for accelerated brain research, but for the availability of all kinds of apps, music and other technology to enhance the effect of your brain waves. I want to emphasize that when we want to have a sharp and alert mind, it is important to access our beta brainwaves, 14-40 Hz. When it is time to rest, it is best when our theta and delta waves are activated in the range of 1-8 Hz. The problem is, in our wired and tired world, we don't often access this powerful part of our brain where we can feel bliss and deep connection. Fortunately meditation, breathing exercises, HeartMath and some of the methods listed below and in Chapter 10 access this part of your brain.

Five Common Brain Waves

Figure 6A clearly outlines our main brain waves with the measurements in Hz—a unit of frequency in the International System of units (SI). It is defined as one cycle per second. Let's take a quick look at some of the different types of brain waves, knowing that they all serve a purpose. Learning to access more of the theta and delta waves will dramatically increase your Healthy Conscious Traveler's Status, as well as your IQ!

Gamma brain waves operate between 30-60 Hz (or cycles per second.) They are the fastest frequencies and are associated with insight, peak concentration and extremely high levels of cognitive functioning. Gamma waves were literally unknown until the advent of digital electroencephalography, since analog electroencephalography could only measure up to around 25 Hz. It's quite interesting that the Gamma wave affects the entire brain. It has a "full sweep" action and creates an inner environment that can translate into peak mental and physical performance.

Beta brain waves are cycling between 14 and 40 Hz. At this level, you would be experiencing a normal waking consciousness that would include a heightened state of alertness. This is where your ability to use logic and critical reasoning comes in. Although this state is necessary for you to carry out your normal daily functions, it can also be a fertile ground for stress and anxiety. Considering the fact that most adults are operating quite consistently at the beta level, it makes sense that stress would be one of today's most common complaints.

Alpha brain waves range between 7.5 and 14 Hz and bring about a state of deep relaxation. With the decrease in brain rhythm, there is a significant increase in the levels of beta-endorphin, norepinephrine and dopamine, the feel-good chemistry of the brain. These waves open the gates to the subconscious and to your intuition. It is important for the HCT to live more in this wave frequency range.

Theta brain waves (see the photo at the beginning of this chapter) that range between 4 and 7.5 Hz can take you to a place of great inspiration. This is where creativity and insight abounds. Although your body is in a deep state of relaxation, it is at the border of the alpha and theta brainwaves that you can visualize and consciously create your reality.

Delta brain waves that range between 1 to 8 Hz are the slowest frequencies and this is where the body goes into deep sleep and the mind is in the dimension of the unconscious. This is the deepest sleep you can have, and it's where deep healing and regeneration take place. These restorative waves slow down the body's metabolism and allow the body to heal both mentally and physically. It is interesting to note that people who display a deep sense of empathy for others produce slower delta waves. This state allows a person to better relate and understand how another person is feeling. When you are in a constant state of stress or in the Red Zone and are out of the Green Zone, you cannot reach this level and are likely to awake from sleep feeling less than fresh and restored.

How Your Brain and Nervous System Are Affected by Negative EMFs

Have you questioned why you often do not feel great after extended periods of time in cars and other forms of transportation? Experts like Debra Davis, a former researcher from the National Academy of Science and the president-founder of the Environmental Health Trust, states: "The effect of negative EMFs and radiation on the brain and other vulnerable tissue is much like snapping a rubber band; snap it once, and it stays intact, but snap it constantly and irregularly, and the rubber band falls apart."(4)

Also, in a University of Washington study, scientists exposed live rats to cell phone radiation and then examined their brains. They found that "DNA from the brains of exposed rats was damaged, while DNA from unexposed rat brains remained intact.(5)

Based on research by filmmaker Talal Jabari's in his documentary film *Full Signal*, the health effects from exposure to high and consistent levels of radiation frequency from industry sources have an astonishing effect on the human body, all the way to its cellular level. In terms of the brain, there is memory loss, inability to learn, inability to sleep, and speech loss. Regular exposure also highly compromises the immune system, making it far more vulnerable to diseases. In addition, women and men are experiencing increasing infertility and impotency. Women's cycles are significantly disrupted when exposed to radiation frequencies. It even affects our DNA. Single and double strands break, which could eventually lead to genetic mutation.

Perhaps Dr. Andrew Weil said it best when he stated that electromagnetic pollution (EMF) may be the worst kind of pollution produced by human activity because it is virtually undetectable as it's invisible and insensible. Following The 8 Pathways in this book is your best defense from EMF pollution.

Moods, Foods, Hormones and Brain Function

One of the ways to access your brain function and to understand your moods is through a comprehensive hormonal test, as well as a blood or urine test. An easy and inexpensive way to understand your moods is to use a mood questionnaire created by Julia Ross, author of *The Mood Cure*. I have also interviewed Trudy Scott, C.N., and recommend her book *The Anti-Anxiety Food Solution*. The interviews with Trudy Scott and Julia Ross are available at www.jointhe selfcarerevolution.com.

To take the mood quiz by Trudy Scott, go to Appendix B in this book now. It takes less than five minutes to fill out. The quiz will help you understand if you are deficient in one of the good mood hormones, called serotonin and dopamine, or if you are lacking in other brain neurotransmitters such as Gaba and norepinephrine. The point here is that in many cases, you can discover what you're missing and immediately start taking supplements that will help you get your nutritional deficiencies handled. Most importantly, you can also begin to eat nourishing foods to correct your deficiencies and excesses.

I am a big fan of both Ross and Scott's books and feel that this quiz alone has helped my patients save thousands of dollars on expensive lab tests. In fact, these are the books I recommend most often to my patients, especially those seeking alternatives to prescription drugs for anxiety and depression. I also direct my patients to the HCT foods and supplements (listed below) that will help them to restore healthy moods, brain function and sleep.

When I first took this quiz years ago, I was deficient in Gaba and dopamine. This is very common for people who are reaching for a cigarette, alcohol or excessive exercise. I fit in the excessive exercise category. For about two decades, I was prone to over-exercise and over-train for my next marathon and thrill-seeking adventure, like jumping out of planes, bungee jumping or exotic travel. Often, people like me are seeking that most addictive "flow state," where we are fully immersed and focused on an activity that brings great pleasure. It's much like a "runner's high," and I find that when I travel, I can easily get into this flow state.

A patient who travels regularly came in to see me with severe brain fog, fatigue and mild depression. Through lab tests, we discovered she had low testosterone and DHEA, high cortisol and suffered from hypothyroidism. She was not moving through life with optimal brain capacity or stress resiliency. Through acupuncture, herbal supplements and a dietary makeover, she was able to get back her clarity, energy and passion for life. She was also able to finally start building muscle from her exercise program.

It is absolutely essential for you, HCT, to find out what is going on with your hormones for healthy travel. Visit your doctor and request a hormone profile via blood or urine. I often recommend the 24-hour urine test from Meridian Valley. To find out more about hormone health, read Sara Gottfried's book, *The Hormone Cure* and her more recent book *The Hormone Reset Diet*.

Multi-tasking

John Medina, author of *Brain Rules*, tells us the brain cannot multi-task, period! What it does do is switch back and forth between tasks very quickly. Medina further says that someone whose attention is interrupted not only takes 50% longer to accomplish a task but also makes up to 50% more errors.(7) A study in *The New England Journal of Medicine* found that people who talk on cell phones while driving are four times more likely to have an accident, because it isn't possible to devote your full attention to both driving and talking at the same time. Hands-free calling offers no advantage. What's the lesson here? Focus on one task at a time, and you'll accomplish each better and faster and without hurting anybody.(8)

Nutrition and fitness for your brain

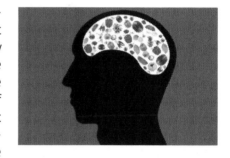

Your brain needs lots of oxygen exchange, and it is most important to have healthy mitochondria, which is where the gasoline or fuel of the body is produced in each of your cells. You definitely want to take good care of your mitochondria! In addition to the excellent food choices already mentioned, consider the following natural supplements. Your brain needs to be fed and tenderly cared for, just like the rest of you. Some consider it even *more* important than certain other aspects of your health.

Brain Sharpener: This is one of my top supplements for brain health. It is a "perfect brain food" that has a combination of herbs, vitamins and other ingredients (many of the ones listed below) that support brain chemistry balance and can lower anxiety and, yes, cortisol. The company that produces it states: "It is the student's best help in taking exams." It aids with neurological well-being, memory restoration, depression, energy and general well-being. Many of my patients find it extremely helpful. (See www.santafesoul.com.)

CoQ10: This supplement can activate enzymes in the mitochondria to produce adenosine triphosphate (ATP), which is our cell's primary energy source. It also acts as an antioxidant to neutralize free radicals that are created when ATP is produced. CoQ10 is an excellent antioxidant choice, and is good for your heart.

D-Ribose: This is a simple five-carbon sugar that the body, instead of burning it, reserves for the work of making ATP. ATP is the energy molecule that powers every tissue in our body. D-Ribose increases energy, improves mental clarity or "brain fog" and encourages the overall feeling of well-being. I highly recommend D-Ribose for everyone who exercises on a regular basis. It helps to remove lactic acid buildup and it is excellent for your heart and circulatory system. D-Ribose is always part of my exercise routine. I just add it to my water.

Acetyl-L-Carnitine: This amino acid has been studied extensively and found to have significant cognitive and anti-aging effects. It is known to be effective for improving mood and one's response to stress as well as lessening memory deficits.

Vitamin B6 (Pyridoxine): This B vitamin is a water-soluble nutrient that helps to calm the nervous system as well as aid in its maintenance. It is essential for the production of neurotransmitters—the brain chemicals that allow the nerve cells to communicate with each other—and plays an important part in the metabolic processes of the body. B6 supplementation is also used to treat memory loss and depression.

Glutathione: This molecule is considered to be the most powerful antioxidant in the body. It protects the mitochondria from bacteria, viruses and toxins. Glutathione is the brain's primary antioxidant. Because the brain generates more oxidative byproducts than any other organ, it is very susceptible to the attack of free radicals. This oxidative stress is an important cause of brain injury and neurodegenerative disease. As we age, our glutathione levels decrease significantly, so its importance as a supplement cannot be overstated. My favorite glutathione product is Tri-Fortify, which is in an absorbable liposomal delivery system. Visit Chapter 9 for more information on this potent antioxidant.

Phosphatidylserine (PS): PS supports memory, judgment, reasoning and neuroplasticity of the brain. It is able to replace damaged neurons and generate new ones. It is truly a building block for your brain's 100 billion nerve cells. Neuroplasticity and communication between neurons depend on a steady supply of PS, and PS is crucial for the prevention of cognitive decline as we age.

Phosphatidylcholine: This is a major chemical messenger for memory, thoughts, focus, and other brain functions. Its bioactive form promotes concentration and builds new cell membrane mass.

Superoxide Dismutase (SOD): We are born with this enzyme, which is responsible for putting out the fire in your body, and more specifically reducing ROS (reactive oxygen species) or free radicals. SOD is a strong antioxidant, and it reduces the amyloid plaque deposits associated with Alzheimer's disease. Some people, like me, do not have enough SOD enzymes (mine are genetically cramped), so I need to take SOD supplements. Having an SOD mutation doesn't necessarily mean you will develop cognitive dysfunction. SOD, as a supplement, provides five critical nutrients to your brain that it craves to stay healthy and alert, all in one tiny and easy-to-swallow "package." Yes, you get this too when you add a daily package of your favorite Oxylent supplement to water.

St. John's Wort: This great herb has long been used medicinally, primarily as an antiseptic, anti-inflammatory and astringent. Interestingly, the herb was first used as a treatment for mental health concerns in ancient Greece, as a remedy for "demonic possession" and "melancholia." It has been used quite effectively for mild to moderate depression. St. John's Wort may not be as effective for more severe cases of depression. It can make your skin more sensitive to the sun, so it may not be the thing for your beach vacation. It is best to check with your physician before using this herb, as there are some safety concerns with certain disorders.

Omega-3 Fats: Your brain is made up of this fat, and deficiency can lead to a host of problems. Supplement with 1,000 to 4,000 mg of purified fish oil a day. Most everyone has heard of the benefits of EPA/DHA fish oils for the brain, alleviating depression and acting as a natural anti-inflammatory agent. *Know* that not all EPA/DHA is made alike. The National Institute of Health (NIH) recommends a daily intake of 650 mg of EPA/DHA for healthy individuals. The omega-3s are found in fish, flax and chia seeds, some eggs and grass-fed butter. Walnuts, sardines, brussel sprouts, kale and spinach may lower blood levels of a problematic protein called beta-amyloid associated with Alzheimer's and other memory problems. (9)

Vitamin D: Deficiency in this essential vitamin can lead to depression, bone loss and increase your incidence of most diseases! Supplement with at least 2,000 to 5,000 IU of vitamin D3 a day. Follow the Healthy Conscious Traveler's Blueprint in Chapter 8 for special pre-trip dosing. I learned from my friend Norm Shealy, M.D., to increase your vitamin D intake up to 50,000 IU for 1-2 days when you feel a cold coming on. This dosing helps prevent a serious infection by stimulating your immune system.

Vitamin B12: Take 1,000 micrograms (mcg) each day as well as B6 25 mgand 800 mcg of folate. These vitamins are critical for metabolizing homocysteine, which can be a factor in depression.

Four important considerations for the HCT

To repeat, nourish yourself regularly with an **anti-inflammatory, elimination diet** that gets rid of common food allergens. As I mentioned above, food allergies and the resultant inflammation have been connected with depression, stress and other mood disorders.

Check for **hypothyroidism, hyperthyroidism and Hashimoto's disease**, a largely unrecognized epidemic that is a leading cause of depression and other health issues. Make sure to have a thorough thyroid exam and blood test if you are depressed and have one or more of the many symptoms associated with thyroid dysfunction. Note that blood tests alone are not accurate for thyroid conditions. Work with a doctor who can assess your current thyroid status to support healthy travel.

Get checked for **mercury, lead and other types of heavy metal toxicity**, which have been linked to depression and other mood and neurological problems. "Doctors Data" is the lab I use. Researcher Dr. Magda Havas, Ph.D., states that heavy metal toxicity also contributes to electro-hypersensitivity and all the effects of electro-smog. (See Chapter 7.)

It is essential, HCT, to increase your **vitamin D** levels. As mentioned above, deficiency in this essential vitamin can lead to depression, bone loss and can increase your incidence of most diseases!

Improve your mental fitness, moods and stress resiliency while traveling

It is important that we continue to grow a healthy brain, like all of our organs. To give your brain its best medicine to further its growth and capacity, try some of these suggestions below.

1. Listen to Music. Music is a powerful healer, especially when it is in the lower brain frequency ranges. For millennia, music has touched the hearts and souls of people all around the globe. Music can actually activate neurons across the corpus callosum, which connects the left and right hemispheres of the brain. Generally speaking, non-vocal music stimulates the right brain and singing stimulates the left hemisphere. Music cannot only stimulate emotions and memories, it also can boost the release of those feel-good endorphins in the brain.

2. Smiling has a huge impact on our immune system. Did you know that smiling stimulates pleasure centers in the brain in such an intense way that you would have to consume 2,000 pounds of chocolate for the equivalent stimulation? Wow! Regular travel is an opportunity for you to practice living in joy without letting the irritations of the unknown wear and tear you down and erode your happiness landscape.

3. Good Foods Plus Supplements to Keep the Brain Sharp. I am an advocate of whole-food supplements whenever possible, but there is nothing like getting your needed nutrients from whole foods. It is important to not over or under dose with supplements. To make sure you are taking the right type and amount, consult your physician or health practitioner.

4. Read or Do Something New Every Day. Novelty enhances your brain function and you often learn something at the same time, which is why many of us love to travel. For sure, my brain gets turned on when I visit ancient sites such as Machu Picchu in Peru, the Pyramids of Egypt or climb the Great Wall of China.

5. Play Brain-Strengthening Games that engage new parts of your brain. Sudoku, crosswords, mazes, brain teasers, and other types of puzzles are all effective ways to challenge your mind. Dr. Daniel Amen says that our brains have the ability to change structure and even its physiology when exposed to new information, puzzles and new stimuli.(10) So try something new and really give your brain a workout. Lumosity is a brain improvement program that uses games to train the brain. It offers challenges that push your brain to operate at increased levels. You can subscribe to become a member or download the free app on your phone or iPad and give your brain a daily workout.

6. Learn about and Practice HeartMath, which is excellent for your heart by creating coherence, and this in turn helps create a healthy brain-heart connection as well as aiding with stress management.

7. Challenge Your Memory and Use Your Powers of Recollection on a Regular Basis. Try to remember what you did the past two Fridays. What month was your last family reunion? What were the highlights of your last cruise? Who was the first person to call you on your last birthday?

Call to action:

- The best antidote to a bad mood is gratitude. Write down three things you are grateful for each day.

- Every day that you are on the road, make sure that you get brain-enhancing physical exercise. Try climbing the stairs to your hotel room rather than using the elevator. While watching the morning news, do some planks, burpees and crunches. You could run in place or turn on some spirited music and dance for a cardio workout.

- If you could have a conversation with your brain, what would it have to say to you and vice versa?

- Write down the following quotes below to snap out of bad moods and reactive behavior while on the road. Get over it asap and blossom instead of contracting when irritated unexpectedly while traveling.

The art of being happy lies in the power of extracting happiness from common things. ~ Henry Ward Beecher

Our deepest fear is not that we are inadequate. Our deepest fear is that we are powerful beyond measure. ~ Marianne Williamson

You are not the thoughts in your head. ~ Eckhart Tolle

"Out of chaos comes order. ~ Nietzsche

Fidelity to the law of your own being is an act of high courage flung in the face of life. ~ Carl Jung

And the day came when the risk to remain tight in a bud was more painful than the risk it took to blossom. ~ Anais Nin

Don't ask yourself what the world needs. Ask yourself what makes you come alive and then go do that. Because what the world needs is people who have come alive. ~ Howard Thurman

The mind is everything. What you think, you become. What you feel, you attract. What you imagine, you create. ~ Buddha

In a gentle way, you can shake the world. ~ Gandhi

To feel successful, you must be able to be honest about the things that are really important to you. ~ Daniel Amen, M.D.

Chapter 7

Travel Advice for the Highly Sensitive and the Electro-hypersensitive Person

They tear up at phone commercials, they brood for days after a gentle ribbing. They know what you are feeling before you do. Their nerve cells are actually hyper-reactive. Say hello to the highly sensitive person—you've probably already made him cry.
~ Andrea Bartz

Why Dedicate a Whole Chapter to the HSP/EHS Person?

A growing number of people worldwide are becoming highly sensitive to crowds, sounds, and environmental toxins. Indoor chemical pollution includes air conditioning, off-gassing from rugs, household cleaning products and pesticides. Electromagnetic frequencies (EMF), electro-smog from Wi-Fi, radio frequencies, beacon signals, radiation exposures from microwaves and a variety of other erratic frequencies are increasing daily.

If you live in this toxic world, you may not even know that you could be suffering from Electro-hypersensitivity (EHS) or Environmental illness (EI), the symptoms of which are commonly experienced by highly sensitive people (HSP).

More and more people are going to their medical doctors or integrative, functional medicine practitioners with symptoms from tremors to palpitations and even gastrointestinal (GI) problems and depression (Figure 7a). These symptoms, which are not only caused by travel, have become increasingly common globally. About 10 to 15 million people have been documented worldwide with Electro-hypersensitivity. These people are "the canaries in the coal mine," as the world continues to expand its use of the technologies that cause these problems.

I was once severely EHS and will always be what is known as an extroverted HSP.

I only discovered this through trying to solve my debilitating, long-term sleep problem, as I shared in Chapter 5. This awareness changed my life, my practice, and my full understanding of how we function on a cellular level. For months and now years, I have researched the effects of electromagnetic and environmental pollution. These are two big health challenges in the travel industry, making this an essential chapter for any HCT to understand, and more importantly to encourage you to take the necessary precautions to protect your own body.

In 2011, the World Health Organization (WHO) declared EHS as a new disease category, adding to the 30,000 already known diseases. Through its international EMF Project, WHO is working to identify research needs and is coordinating a worldwide program of EMF studies to allow a better understanding of health risks associated with EMF exposure. Particular emphasis is placed on possible health consequences of low-level EMF. Information about the EMF Project and EMF effects is provided in a series of fact sheets in several languages available at the WHO.(1)

Sweden has classified Electro-hypersensitivity as a disability, and provides its citizens with health care facilities that offer lower levels of exposure to electromagnetic fields and radiofrequency radiation. Additionally, the Canadian Human Rights Commission Report also acknowledges environmental sensitivity attributed to electromagnetic exposure. The report estimates that 3% of the population has severe symptoms of EHS, while another 35% of the population has moderate symptoms, including an impaired immune system and chronic illness. Other countries including Italy, Austria, Norway, Brazil, Germany and Finland, have taken declaration initiatives.(3)

ELECTRO-HYPERSENSITIVITY:

W.H.O. DISEASE CATEGORY

WORLD WIDE!!

Symptoms:

GI problems, sleep problems, fear, stress, hormone imbalance, virus/toxin overload, cataracts, ear ringing, skin rashes, joint pain and tremors, headaches and fatigue, memory loss and confusion, depression, attention deficit...

Figure 7A

A good number of my patients, including flight attendants and pilots who have worked in the travel industry for years, agree that they have become more hypersensitive to certain smells, sounds, long air travel and lighting. Being in an enclosed area can become increasingly uncomfortable and even unbearable at times. Every minute you are in an airplane, you are exposed to solar and cosmic radiation, compounded by radiation exposure from the actual electromagnetic frequencies emanating from the plane. A pilot confided in me that when the solar flares are intense, he drops the plane down 10 feet to protect himself as well as the passengers. Other exposures include flame retardants, pesticides, airplane fuel, and toxic perfumes worn by passengers.

One of my patients worked as a flight attendant for 32 years and started to develop fibromyalgia, sleep disturbances and restless leg syndrome within a few years of starting her job. Each year her symptoms grew worse until she finally accepted early retirement because, as she said, "I could not stand working another month when I could barely push a travel bag under the seat without excruciating pain."

As our bodies continue to be saturated by these artificial frequencies and toxins, the body's ability to take in energy and detoxify becomes compromised. The normal operating system in our bodies becomes overwhelmed and challenged, and we develop symptoms we have never had before. It's time that we think about the health of our body in a completely different way!

Since I have researched EMFs for years, I have become a better health detective. When people come to me for help when all else has failed, I can often determine a connection to EMF exposure. Sometimes all it takes is for people to turn off their Wi-Fi at night to restore restlessness, heart palpitations and migraine headaches.

To clarify, a highly sensitive person (HSP) is someone who has a finely-tuned nervous system, is often detail-oriented, and is extremely intuitive and highly conscientious. Psychologist Carl Jung said such people are naturally more influenced by their unconscious, which gives them information of the "utmost importance," even a "prophetic foresight." Jung further said that even though a life lived in deep communication can be influential and satisfying, it can also be potentially more difficult.

In her book *The Highly Sensitive Person*, Dr. Elaine Aron shares that HSPs are the visionaries, writers, historians, philosophers, artists, teachers, healers and are "plain conscientious citizens."(4)

Are you an HSP?

HSP ASSESSMENT QUESTIONNAIRE

Let's identify whether you are an HSP. Rate your answers to these questions with a number from 1 to 10, 1 being not relevant at all, 5 somewhat relevant, and 10 most relevant.

HSP Assessment Questions	(1-10)
Do you feel a sense of overload when in social settings?	

Are you overly sensitive to certain smells, sounds, fabrics, foods or places?	
Are you hypersensitive regarding your space and your boundaries?	
Do you sense "things" about situations or people that others typically don't?	
Do you feel severely overwhelmed by life, to the point of panic?	
Are you seen as an overly emotional, sensitive, intellectual person?	
Are you overly conscientious of everything you do or say?	
Are you sensitive to low, high or erratic electromagnetic frequencies?	
Do you experience physical, mental, or emotional exhaustion after meeting new people or visiting new places, to the point where you need to isolate in order to release and recharge?	
Are you hypersensitive to pharmaceutical drugs, herbs and supplements?	
Total Score: < 30 average sensitivity > 30 mild HSP > 50 severe HSP	

If your total was higher than 30, you need to keep reading.

Challenges of HSPs

A great deal of HSP conditions are misdiagnosed or mistreated, and therefore, it is critical that you become not only self-aware but self-educated. This allows you to identify, articulate and address your condition more effectively and to find the right health provider to help you move into the Green zone.

The nervous system of the HSP is set to register stimuli at a very low frequency and to amplify it internally. The HSP is much more sensitive to artificial frequencies, which are invisible, and most people are unaware of them. For example, the HSP may not be able to walk into shopping malls, movie theaters, cafes or performance centers because of the noise. EMF and light pollution could instantly cause headaches, vertigo and even palpitations. I see more and more patients each year with this challenge.

HSPs have a complex inner life and need time to process the constant flow of sensory and auditory data. They need more time than most to assimilate acute infections, traumas or stressful events.

HSPs have a low threshold for sensory input and pain and are much more sensitive to toxic fumes and mold exposure. Most HSPs will avoid nail salons, move out of their home during renovations, and get sick as soon as pesticides are used and cannot tolerate petroleum candles. Is this you? These symptoms are most common with people who live 24/7 in the Red Zone and even with HSPs in the Yellow Zone. (See chapters 1 and 8.)

Social interactions can give HSPs the highest highs and the lowest lows. They have a lower threshold of activation of stress hormones that leave the body flooded with cortisol and adrenaline. When left unchecked, these overactive hormones influence adverse changes in the physiology of the body, including increased heart rate, memory loss, confusion, palpitations, vertigo and the like. Also, higher sustained levels of cortisol (as discussed in chapters 5 and 6) often lead to sleep problems, anxiety, high acidity in the blood, weight gain and many other symptoms.

HSPs can also experience a myriad of symptoms that don't seem to have a root cause, however, early childhood trauma is common, but when properly assessed, the source of the health conditions become known so that they can be managed or resolved effectively with self-care tools such as meditation, self hypnosis, tapping and movement. (See chapters 8 and 10.)

Recently, I have noticed in my practice that there has been a real increase in the number of patients dealing with multiple chemical sensitivities (MCS) and EHS symptoms and are generally highly sensitive people (HSP). Know that if you are living in a chronic state of stress in the Red Zone, you need to be vigilant to turn this all around.

Susceptibilities of HSP

Nervous System	Physical	Sensory	Social
Fight /Flight	Skin irritations	Overload input	Over-stimulation
Adrenal excess	Sleeplessness	Light sensitivity	Anxiety
Cortisol excess	Weight gain	Ear ringing	Nervousness
Low cortisol	Deep fatigue	Feeling shaky	Withdrawal
Low dopamine	Insulin peaks, addiction	Sound irritation	Moodiness
Low serotonin	Pain, depression	Smell sensitivity	Overwhelm
Low blood sugar	Tremors	Eye sensitivity	Easily angered

Contributing Factors for HSP

Electro-smog (cell phones, Wi-Fi, etc.)	Social Stimuli (crowds, noise)	Neurological Stimuli (sound, smell)	Food/ Chemical Allergies

You've already learned in Chapter 1 that, much like traffic lights, you have either come to a full stop (Red Zone-Chronic Health Challenge) and you may or may not be aware of the reality of your health crisis and what to do about it, or you have come to a cautious place (Yellow), where you are aware of your healthy challenges but remain stuck in adverse patterns that are hard to change, or you have claimed responsibility for your health choices and are living a self-care, highly functioning lifestyle (Green). When you're living in the Green Zone, you are riding the open highway of optimum vitality.

By now, you have established whether you are an HSP and have identified with either the Red, Yellow or Green field. Let's do a quick assessment. Just circle the areas below that most relate to you.

RED	YELLOW	GREEN
Anxiety/depression	Semi-healthy diet	Restful sleep
Skin problems/ dis-ease	Stress management	Healthy diet
Sleeplessness	Out of balance	Stress free, clarity
Irritability (wired and tired)	Indigestion	Balanced lifestyle
Digestive issues	Food allergies	Proper digestion
Blood sugar issues	Chemical intolerance	Strong immune system
Unhealthy diet	Brain fog	Personal responsibility
Sensory overload	Low energy	Presence/ sustainability
Fight or flight response	Some social anxiety	Love life/ passion-filled
Living by default/ a YES person	Life is just OK	Living by design/ can say no, good boundaries
Score:	Score:	Score:

If you scored higher in the Yellow and Red fields, let's take a look at how to best support your health. If you scored high on the Green, then you are well on your way to optimum health and this book will only support and empower you to continue on that path. Let's look at the following action steps for each of the HCT traffic lights.

For the Reds, eventual breakdown! I highly advise the following action steps:

Get immediate help from a qualified practitioner who will conduct a thorough evaluation including a blood, stool, heavy metal and adrenal testing, *not* just a clinician who is going to give you prescription drugs. Your body is crying for some serious attention to bring it out of this "fight or flight" stress state.

It's high time to make some significant lifestyle changes.

Decide what are your stressors in life (work, toxic relationships, etc.) and know which ones you are able to eliminate. Chronic dehydration is also a big stressor, so make sure you are properly hydrated daily.

Electro-sanitize your home and office immediately. Turn off your Wi-Fi at night, take breaks from your computer and unplug all appliances that are not necessary within six feet of where you sleep. Refer to Chapter 8 for how to effectively electro-sanitize your home/office/travel and how to best support your immune system while traveling.

Spend time outside connecting with energy through Earthing (Vitamin E for Earthing), grounding or simply walking outside for 20 minutes every day.

Amp up your healthy diet by adding high-voltage foods, such as organic fruits and veggies, grass-fed beef, nuts, berries and other living foods that come directly from the earth.

For the Yellows, I encourage the following action steps:

I would suggest the same directives as the Red, but maybe not as urgently. You are receiving alarms that your body is not functioning optimally and change is needed. Perhaps it's time for a detox program and to support your body with adaptogenic vitamins and herbs.(See Chapter 9.) As mentioned above, make sure you are properly hydrated daily and getting enough rest.

I highly encourage you get the tests done that are recommended in the Red category so you can be evaluated and avoid ever being in the Red Zone.

Also, it's time to clean up your diet so you're only eating natural, organic, living foods that support your body, instead of foods that are making you sick, as processed foods do.

For the Greens, here are some pointers that will help you strengthen your awesome commitment to yourself:

Keep up your self-care lifestyle knowing that, as I always say to my patients, "self-care is a way of life, not an event."

Amp up your healthy diet by adding high-voltage foods such as organic fruits and veggies, grass-fed beef, nuts, berries and other living foods that come directly from the earth.

Self-care for the HSP

Many medical conditions arise during short- or long-distance travel that an HSP might be more susceptible to, including jet lag, dehydration, dizziness, ear pain and more. If you suffer from dizziness, one of the most common health problems on planes, you might try putting your head between your knees to increase blood flow to the brain. The risk factors for dizziness include dehydration, oxygen deficiency, sitting for a long period of time, drinking alcohol and some medications for high blood pressure like beta-adrenergic blockers.

You could experience ear pain due to the rapid change in air pressure in the cabin. This disturbs the balance of pressure between the outer ear and the middle ear. Many people feel pain when the higher pressure stretches the eardrum. The eustachian tube, which connects the middle ear to the back of the nose and throat, helps equalize the pressure on the eardrum and causes that welcome pop you feel when the balance is restored. You can help the process by swallowing, chewing gum, yawning, or opening your mouth wide. Or, try a trick known as the Valsalva Maneuver: using your thumb and index finger, pinch your nose closed and exhale, through your closed mouth.

Entering new time zones can be challenging, especially when you cross the international date line. It's best to change the time on your wristwatch to your new time zone and synchronize your sleeping and eating schedules to your new time zone by staying awake until the local bedtime. As mentioned in Chapter 5, expose yourself to natural outdoor light as soon as possible to adapt to your new time zone and reset the circadian rhythms of your body more quickly.

If you are an HCT who is also an HSP, it is critical to take time to create healthy boundaries in every aspect of your life. Thoroughly assess the quality of your life and your time at home and at work and particularly while traveling so you can properly support yourself. Stabilize yourself with the free healing available from taking a walk in the park, doing a few minutes of breath work or meditation, relaxing on the grass or taking a nap at the beach. Take advantage of any outlet that reconnects you to the magnetic frequency of the earth.

Another way to deeply support yourself is to arrive at the airport at least a half hour earlier than recommended, to avoid the adrenaline and cortisol rush of last-minute travel plans.

Preventative protocol for the HSP

See Chapters 8, 9 and 10 for additional information on these items.

Electro-sanitizing Devices	Healing Techniques	Supportive Foods/H$_2$0
1. Micro-current 2. PEMF devices 3. Schumann generator 4. Bioelectric shields 5. Stetzerizers 6. Ionizing crystal lamps 7. Neutralizer stickers 8. Functional clothing	1. Energy medicine 2. Tapping 3. EMDR 4. Prayer/ affirmation 5. Acupuncture 6. Reiki 7. Chiropractic 8. Homeopathy 9. Breathwork 10. Yoga	1. High-voltage foods-live foods from the earth 2. Alkaline water 3. Photonic – structured water 4. Essential oils 5. See HCT-recommended diet in Chap. 2

Not to be repetitive, but I cannot overstate the importance of hydration! Be vigilant and hydrate before, during and after your flight. Drink water with minerals, morning, noon and night!

Become a strong advocate of wholesome nutrition. After all, strong nutrition is the key to your optimum health, especially when you travel often. This ensures optimal cell function and, yes, this is the essence of vibrant health.

WHAT KIND OF SUPPORT DO YOU NEED IF YOU ARE AN HSP?

In my years of practice (and being an HSP) I have worked with many HSPs and people who have endured years of chronic debilitating symptoms that were not properly diagnosed by their doctors. My protocol is to first identify whether the person is an HSP with the following steps:

My first step is to do a thorough medical evaluation in order to identify and treat any specific conditions that may be responsible for the symptoms. I address my patient's overall nutritional habits, hormones, immune system, digestive health (including parasites), nervous system and toxicity levels.

Next I evaluate and identify any psychological conditions that may be responsible for symptoms. I have my patients talk about any problems in their home or work life, any history of mental illness or other problems that might not be readily apparent.

Then I have my patients assess their workplace and home for factors that might contribute to the presented symptoms, including indoor air pollution, excessive noise, poor lighting or flickering light and ergonomic factors. A reduction of stress and other improvements in the work situation might be appropriate.

I have used this approach in my practice for years, and it has not only helped people reclaim their health and to get off their synthetic drugs when possible, but it has empowered my HSP people in particular to make daily choices that promote mood elevation and depression-free lives and to actually know what "feeling good" feels like.

I respectfully dedicate this chapter to all the flight attendants, TSA agents, pilots, ground crew, air traffic controllers, frequent fliers and those who work in the transportation business on a day-to-day basis. I can say, for sure, that not one of my frequent-flying clients always loves the travel part of their job. Complaints abound, like "I feel tired all the time" or "I am out of sync with life" or "My sleep patterns are never normal."

It is important for each of you to know that you are not crazy, that you are not depressed due to a genetic predisposition, and that the industry in which you live and work and the travel choices you make *are* contributing to the unrest you feel inside. The good news is that, as the HCT, you have endless choices and strategies to use daily to keep yourself in the happy, healthy green zone.

Call to action:

• Before you do anything else, go to www.antennasearch.com and type in your address to find out how many cell towers are near your home.

- Support the Frank R. Lautenberg Chemical Safety Bill for the 21st Century Act that will help the Environmental Protection Agency regulate or remove hazardous chemicals from the marketplace—even asbestos, arsenic, chromium, formaldehyde, BPA or other dangerous substances that have been linked to birth defects and cancer.

- To learn more about HSPs and a supportive online groups for HSPs, go to http://www.hsphealth.com/hsp-health-reinvented/HSP.

- Electro-sanitize your home and work environment each day.

- Follow the Red and Yellow suggestions in this chapter to increase your stress resiliency and to feel more joy and less overwhelm.

- Always wear your protective EMF devices on your phone and use your bioelectric shield 24/7. (See Chapter 10.)

- Keep a travel journal, especially if this chapter spoke to you. Create travel rituals to avoid any unforeseen stress that you can prevent. For example, take your own travel comfort foods, pillow and always be at the airport comfortably in advance, to avoid unnecessary stress.

Chapter 8

Generate Your Healthy Travel Blueprint

Proper Preparation Prevents Poor Performance ~ Charlie Batch

Based on Chapter 7, you may have identified yourself as a Highly Sensitive Person (HSP) or one with Electro-hypersensitivity (EHS) or both. As a result of reading this and making positive choices, I trust that you are moving from Red to bright Yellow and hopefully to Green, in terms of your commitment to The 8 Pathways!

Your commitment now lies in generating your healthy travel blueprint, a blueprint that will serve as a navigational tool for preparing yourself for travel and for optimum healthy living. Look at this chapter as your map, and use it to set your confident self on course for the best possible travel experience, each and every time!

The Mindset of the HCT

Follow The 8 Pathways

Elevate your journey to one that is relaxed and effortless by following these pathways to ensure that your trip does not end up being your catch-up time. People often say that it takes them three days to just settle into their five-to-seven day vacation.

Develop the mindset of whole-life travel that supports body, mind and spirit.

Embody the conscious travel mantra: *I am an energized, fit, smart and conscious traveler.*

Whenever possible, completely unplug from all electronics, enjoy every sunset and every moment of stillness.

Create time for fun and games, dance and sunset-gazing—no wristwatch. In fact, maybe leave your watch at home, especially if it is leisure travel.

Spend time at the beach or other nature spots and soak up the sun's rays, which offer the best frequencies ever. Go "barefooting" whenever possible.

Nurture your creativity, journal, and take long walks to explore new territory.

Go for the GREEN Lifestyle Each Day for Healthy Traveling (as seen in Chapter 7 and modified here for the Healthy Travel Blueprint! Circle the descriptions that apply to you.

RED	YELLOW	GREEN
Unhealthy diet	Semi-healthy diet	Healthy diet
Fight or flight response	Stress management	Managing stress well
Sleeplessness	Fitful sleep	Restful sleep
Regular digestive issues	Indigestion	Proper digestion
Sensory overload	Mild brain fog	Presence/ sustainability
Living by default	Life is status quo	Living by design
Anxiety/depression	Moodiness/feeling edgy	Maintaining positive moods
Irritability (wired and tired)	Apathy	Love for life/ passion-filled
Disease/weak immune system	Occasional illness	Strong immune system

"Yes" person, no boundaries	Some boundaries	Strong personal boundaries, saying NO is easy
Total lethargy	Low energy	Vibrant living
Highly allergic to food	Food sensitivities	Allergy-free
Blood sugar issues	Moderate sugar imbalance	Balanced sugar levels
Reactive	Semi-reactive	Personal responsibility
Overwhelmed	Adaptable	Resilient
Chemically intolerant	Chemically sensitive	Non-reactive
Severe skin problems	Mild skin reactions	Non-reactive
Score:	Score:	Score:

If you score high in the Red and Yellow, it is important to make lifestyle changes as soon as possible. If you score high on the Green, then you are well on your way to optimum health, and this book will support and empower you to continue on that path. Let's look at the following action steps for each of the HCT traffic lights.

For the REDS: I highly advise the following action steps. Consider working with a holistic health practitioner as soon as possible to assess your overall health. I would highly recommend comprehensive blood work, food allergy/sensitivity tests, adrenal saliva test and heavy metal tests. Eat a healthy plant-based diet, including grass-fed meat, if not vegetarian. Make sure you are taking the Core 6 Supplements (see below), and that you are drinking enough water and exercising at least three times a week. Take restorative rest days to recharge your body. Learn to say "no" to all the demands on your life that are not essential, and unplug from technology as often as possible.

For the YELLOWS: Go for a cleaner diet as part of your Healthy Conscious Traveler blueprint, say "no" more often and spend more time outdoors. Try to complete items on your to-do list, meditate more and see what two things you can do today to foster more checks in the Green Zone.

For the GREENS: Keep up the good work! Here are some pointers that will help you remain in the Green Zone. Take time to reflect on the benefits of your self-care lifestyle and notice how much more you can do and *be* when in this zone. Be proactive in the moment to continually make choices that keep you in the Green Zone, especially if you travel often. Positive actions compounded over time equals sustained, optimal health. Congrats to you for accomplishing a level of health that few realize in today's world!

How to Best Support Yourself Prior to Travel

Forewarned, forearmed; to be prepared is half the victory.
~ Miguel de Cervantes

Getting Ready: This is one of the most important aspects of any trip you might take. Here are some ideas, tips and suggestions that will allow you to have a more enjoyable and healthier experience; i.e., how to survive travel in comfort and style.

Set Your Travel Intention: The law of attraction is at play here. When you are prepared and ready to have a wonderful trip, you are more likely to attract what you want rather than when you are exhausted and running around like crazy, trying to get everything done at the last minute. Ask yourself, "What is my intention for this trip?" (Pathway 7). Clarity will bring you ease and strength.

Logistics: Create a checklist for getting your travel documents together. Arrange for house, plants, pet sitters, emergency contacts, vaccinations, passport/visa, driver's license or other proper identification. Aim to be in the Yellow to Green zones well before your trip to enjoy your travels and to minimize stress all around (Pathway 7).

Planning: Start packing one week prior to departure! Also, start researching your most eco-friendly options, like low-EMF cars, non-smoking, toxic-free rooms, and first-floor hotel rooms. Yes, sleeping closer to the ground is a better choice, as the increased positive charge on upper floors can affect those whose health is already poor. In times past, humans slept on the ground, in touch with subtle energy from the earth. Recent research has revealed an up-lifting shift in our physiology.(1) So I say, closer to the ground is best! Also stay away from hotel rooms on floors where all the con-ferences are due to the increase of electronics and noise.

Brain and Energy Medicine Strategies: Use the emotional free-dom technique (EFT), self-hypnosis, acupressure and visualization (see Chapter 10) to clear any blocks to a successful trip. At night, clear your head and visualize and feel exactly how you want to see your trip unfold. Visualize your flights leaving on time, light traffic and getting to your destination in a timely manner.

Culture and Customs: Educate yourself about your destination prior to your trip, and research the area you will be visiting to get familiarized with the language, tipping customs, and social and dress etiquette. For example, in many developing nations, including Haiti and Guatemala, girls and women mostly wear dresses. Female tourists are expected to respect this code. When I was in Haiti, all the women in my group were asked to follow the dress code. I am a runner, so when it was time for me to do my daily run, guess what? I ran in my skirt. You can imagine the looks I got!

This is especially important during cultural events in certain countries. I was in Bhutan on the day a new king was crowned. We attended this special event by dressing in the Bhutanese ceremo-nial dress. It was one of the most colorful and memorable travel days of my life!

Refrigerator: Make sure your hotel room has a refrigerator for food you will be taking with you or buying along the way. Most hotels can arrange to put one in your room at the same time that you make your travel arrange-ments, sometimes for an additional fee. If you are traveling by car, pack a few small coolers, including a foldable version. Attending to this one item will make your food choices so much easier.

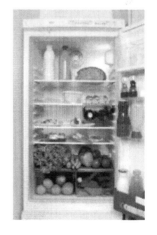

Health Protocols: Get your neck ad-justed if necessary. A massage before a trip is a great choice. Get your bangs cut or mustache trimmed. Go in for a dental checkup if you are due. Fill up on any nec-essary prescriptions or supplements. If you have a health condition, please make sure you have a thorough exam before travel, including a blood test. It is highly recommended that all people who travel regularly get an annual exam.

Prepare your immune system for one month prior to long-distance travel

Four Weeks before You Travel: Practice The 8 Pathways, as always, and consume one green drink per day. Take the top vitamins recommended in Chapter 9 and start planning your trip. Remember your health is not just your wealth but also your state of mind and happiness. Be consistent with healthy choices (Pathway 1).

Three Weeks before You Travel: Continue as above, plus make sure your diet is super clean and free of unnecessary sugar. Look at your schedule and eliminate all activity that is not essential. Add lemon juice to your water each morning to optimize liver function, to clean your lymph system and to alkalinize your blood. Meditate, stretch and make sure you are taking the top 6 supplements.

Two Weeks before You Travel: Continue with suggestions for the weeks prior, plus start adding four grams of vitamin C and other antioxidants (vitamins A, D, Selenium, NAC), as well as increasing your green drink to twice per day. Continue adding lemon juice to your water. This not only increases the energy and voltage of your body but is a boost to your immune system. Be consistent.

One Week before You Travel: Your health is your #1 priority the week before you travel. Increase the amount of fresh organic fruits and vegetables, focusing on a wide variety of all colors of the rainbow. Consume an anti-inflammatory diet (see Chapter 2). Get eight to nine hours of sleep per night (see Chapter 5). Continue with your green drinks, multivitamin, four grams of vitamin C, two to three grams of the essential fatty acids (EFAs) and five 10,000 International Units (IUs) of vitamin D. Also add liquid iodine (good topically and for use in a neti pot, and to detox) and 6 to 12 mg a day of Astaxanthin to protect yourself from radiation. Make sure you are getting at least 30 mg of zinc a day.

It's very important to course-correct when anything is getting in the way of your extreme self-care this week. Start taking .3 to 3 grams of melatonin four days before departure, if traveling internationally. You may find this is one of your sleep supplements of choice on and off throughout the year.

Vaccination Checklist: The Center for Disease Control has an extensive website with travel-related information at http://www. cdc.gov/travel/index.htm. You can check each country's guidelines to find out what vaccinations are required for entry. For example, I was not able to enter Kenya without the yellow fever vaccination. In many parts of the world where malaria is known to occur, such as sub-Saharan Africa, preventative medication is recommended. Do you know that there are homeopathic and Chinese medicine alternative choices to vaccines? Do your vaccine homework to make the best decision for your body, your age and any health history concerns you may have. If the HCT blueprint is followed and necessary preventative steps are taken, these illnesses may be successfully avoided.

This information is provided to keep you safe and healthy during the trip. Please review this guide for detailed health care information and consult with your doctor for the approach that is best for you. Also consider consulting www.healthytraveler.com, a premiere Los Angeles travel medicine clinic for affordable yellow fever immunizations, vaccinations, shots, medicine and consultation.

Mosquito Protection: Almost all commercial insect repellents contain DEET (N,N-diethyl-m-toluamide), which is an effective, yet toxic, insect repellent. Other effective and more natural, options include Buzz Away made by Quantum, Herbal Armor made by All Terrain and Herbal Insect Repellent made by All Around the World. These all contain some combination of eucalyptus, lemongrass, citronella, peppermint, cedar, lavender, and other essential oils. Oral doses of garlic and onion, as well as vitamins B6 and B12 can also be useful in keeping mosquitoes away. Remember to keep your vitamin C intake high with four to six grams per day.

Your Healthy Conscious Traveler's self-care kit

You might want your rosary, your Bible, *The Course in Miracles* book or anything else that gives you comfort. Perhaps a picture of your children or partner to help you relax more deeply while traveling—or maybe not; that's up to you. Many people travel with portable altars.

Take a small bag of your most precious lotions and potions. Coconut oil, cacao oil and butter, lavender oil, tiger balm; there are so many good choices! Truth be told, some of my HCT friends take more of these self-care items than clothes!

Bring an extra copy of your passport, or take a digital copy of your passport, as well as a list of important phone numbers.

Women may want to carry a whistle in their pocket when traveling alone.

Here are some essentials items to include in your traveler's self-care kit. For additional information on medicinal herbs, supplements and super foods, please refer to Chapter 9.

Herbs

Ginger tea for optimum circulation

Chloroxygen for increased red blood cells and improved cellular oxygen

Super foods

David Wolfe's Favorite Super foods. Super Herbs (Greens, Acai berries, Camu Camu, Cacao) and much more (LongevityWarehouse.com)

Supplements (more in Chapter 9)

Oscillococcinum: This homeopathic remedy helps prevent flu symptoms

Aerobic 07 Drops: For increased cellular oxygen levels

Cell Food Drops: For optimum trace minerals, amino acids and enzymes

Hyposcorbate vitamin C from Progena: 4 grams of vitamin C/ serving for supporting a strong immune system

Liquid iodine: good topically and for use in a neti pot and to detox

Astaxanthin: 6 to 12 mg/day to protect yourself from radiation

Zinc: 30mg/day

First-Aid Kit

Keep a small first-aid kit at all times in your luggage. You can find these at all drug stores. Add specialty items, such as homeopathic Arnica Montana for bruising, swelling or muscular pain. You may want to include an over-the-counter medication that you use on occasion, like Neosporin. Homeopathic medicines such as Carbo Vegetabilis or Boiron's Gasalia for painful digestive gas or Nux Vomica for digestive upsets are good to keep in your first-aid kit. My friend, Harmony, travels with activated charcoal and curing pills, just in case of food poisoning. It really saved her from turning inside out when she ate a raw salad in Ecuador. Prep your first-aid kit with Thieves Oil from Young Living Essential Oils and other great oils (www.ylwebsite.com/robynbenson/home) that you can buy at cost by setting up your own account.

Check Out *The Healthy Conscious Traveler's First-Aid Kit* at www. robynbenson.com.

Extra considerations for the frequent traveler

Extra cash, calling card, lip moisturizer, nail clippers, nose and eyebrow tweezers, hand lotion and eye drops (for dry and itchy eyes; Similasan is a great choice).

Water Bottle (BPA-free)

Be sure to keep plastic bottles and food storage containers from heating or extreme cold, as these changes in temperature contribute to the leaking of estrogen-like and other hazardous chemicals into the food/liquid and thus into our bodies. BPA-free water bottles are the best choice. BPA, also known as "Bisphenol A," is a reactive chemical and it mimics the effects of the estrogen hormone. It is a known hormone disruptor. Bisphenol A has been used in all sorts of plastics and resins since 1957, and studies show there is a long list of specific health ailments related to BPA. The list includes: obesity, heart disease, neurological disorders, hyperactivity, attention deficit disorders, propensity for drug abuse, thyroid disorders, breast, brain, and prostate cancers, and reproductive disorders.(2)

Also, to find healthy water during your travels, use Findaspring (http://www.findaspring.com), a community-created database and map of natural spring water sources all over the world!

Compass, GPS System and Maps

Finding your destination with ease is great for your healthy nervous system! Any stress quickly takes away from your travel pleasure. Again, with proper planning you can avoid unnecessary stress and frustration.

Magic Bullet or the Larger Nutri Bullet

If you are one of the growing population of green, fruit and protein smoothie lovers, invest in a small portable blender such as the

Magic Bullet or the larger Nutri Bullet or a simple shake container offered at health food stores that you can pack in your checked luggage. The Magic Bullet blender is handy, versatile and so easy to use that you'll put it to work EVERY single day (probably several times a day). Best of all, it saves you time because it does almost any job in the kitchen in 10 seconds or less! It is great for travel so you can make your own smoothies, juices and more (http://www. buythebullet.com/howitworks.php).

Smoothies

You need some great food for that Nutri-Bullet! Prepare your protein-shake dry goods ahead of time for the days you are away. You can also pack fresh fruits and veggies that can last a few days, or shop when you arrive at your destination.

Travel Pillow for Plane, Train, Bus, Car

I am a huge proponent of pillows that support your neck. Travel and unfamiliar pillows can lead to stiff necks, shoulders and headaches. For the past 10 years, I have traveled with my favorite Tempur Pedic travel pillow (http://www.tempurpedic.com/Travel/ Tempur-Pedic-TravelPillow.asp). It is always in my suitcase ready to go! The wrap-around shape of this travel pillow cradles your neck and supports your head, relieving pressure and letting your neck and shoulder muscles relax. You'll sleep better. This is a great investment to make, supporting your neck during long-distance travel.

Yon Smart Blanket

This smart device is perfect for the traveler. It's a wearable blanket that slips on so it stays in place and gives you mobility while you snuggle up. You can sleep during your flight with privacy, and when you arrive, within seconds you can pack the blanket away in its own carrier pouch. Get it here at www.yonsmartblanket.com.

No matter what your age, a blanket can be your perfect security item to keep you warm while traveling or to snuggle with at night.

Music and Meditation

Bring along your best meditation and relaxation music on your iPod or MP3 player. If you are EHS, HSP or have a short fuse, consider investing in a hypnosis session with a reputable therapist.

Ask to receive a copy of your session that will bring you back into that wonderful sanctuary where you are calm, at peace and not affected by the noise (like snoring) around you while you travel. Also, you can download free apps called "Ambient," "Zen Mixer" and "Remindfulness" from your iPhone app store.

*Healthy conscious traveler's food kit for on the road (*www.robynbenson.com*)*

Consume oxygen and antioxidant-rich foods with a high water content. That would include a variety of greens, vegetables and fruits. Stock up on live organic foods to snack on during your travel day.

Often we find ourselves in places where there are no healthy restaurants or food stores, so plan ahead!

Some of my favorite choices are dried kale, gluten-free pretzels, grass-fed beef, buffalo or salmon jerky, canned sardines and tuna or oysters (much to the chagrin of some of my fellow travelers). My favorite brand of canned and packaged fish is Vital Choice, owned by my super-conscious friend, Randy Hartnell. Get your discount here: www.vitalchoice.com/HealthyTraveler. Super yummy!

Extra nuts, seeds, shredded coconut and boxed coconut water are also good choices. It is prudent to take a little eco-friendly bag of your favorite sea salt and cinnamon for supporting hydration, your immune system and healthy blood sugar levels. Choose stevia as your sweetener. Coconut oil is a must! This can be your body lotion, an emergency hit of healthy saturated fat when you feel deep hunger, and it is always handy for cooking. It is considered to be a cure for many pathogens such as fungus, parasites and other bacteria. I recommend that most people consume two tablespoons per day and use it often in cooking. Coconut oil is one of your best oil choices to sustain your healthy cell membrane walls, which are at least 50% fat! As we know from Bruce Lipton and other scientists, a healthy cell membrane is one of the best indicators of health.

Food Checklist

Take along enough food for 48 hours as part of your HCT Blueprint. This is a great list for your consideration, and it is always good to have on hand for a four-day conference or for pleasure travel too.

- Vital Choice Brand wild albacore tuna (has six times more omega-3 and is low in mercury), sockeye salmon, sardines and salmon jerky. Or make your own jerky.
- A small bag of chia, hemp or flax seeds is full of beneficial nutrients and crunch and can be added easily to Greek yogurt, salad or hot cereal.
- A bag of kale chips
- Three hard-boiled eggs or chicken that you can easily put in a small foldable cooler in your carry-on
- Beef, buffalo, turkey, salmon or tuna jerky—make sure to buy the best quality that is not loaded with additives.
- Two to four whole-food energy bars. Self-care Revolution bars are a great choice (www.jointheselfcarerevolution.com).
- Three pieces of fruit with lower sugar content, such as an apple, pear and orange
- Whole raw almonds, pecans and other nuts of your choice. Avoid peanuts, which are often allergenic and are prone to contamination with aflatoxin and other toxins.
- Gluten-free pretzels
- A small container of sea salt or Bragg's Aminos in powder form
- Coconut oil
- Stevia

If traveling by plane, the extra $30 you spend to take another piece of luggage full of food and snacks saves you from having to buy unhealthy meals for two to four days. Also, you have luggage in which to take home extra clothes, souvenirs and folders from any workshops you might have attended.

The Core 6 Supplements

- A Multivitamin/Mineral(with 30 mg zinc)
- Magnesium (600 mg)
- Probiotics

- Extra vitamin C (4,000 mg/day)
- Vitamin D3 (at least 2,000 - 5,000 IU/ day)
- B-complex

Packing: Here is the packing list I use for my frequent travels. A checklist like this will help make your travel stress-free. Please modify your own list, as you may want to add or delete items that you need or want on your various journeys. Remember to pack in advance. If you are a frequent traveler, always have the basics ready to go, so you can leave at any time. Here's a helpful suggestion: use a list application on your smartphone, or laminate your list and always have it handy.

Your list could include:

- Silverware or an eco-friendly equivalent
- Gauss meter, is a tool to measure magnetic fields and EMF pollution (see Chapter 10.)
- Empty BPA-free container (for smoothies and water)
- Travel mug for your hot beverages
- Clothing, etc.
- Toiletries
- Vitamins, supplements and prescription meds
- Boiron homeopathic medicine for digestive gas
- Earplugs
- Outdoor adventure: hats, gloves, sport or camping equipment, hiking boots
- Bathing suit and PABA-free sun block
- Computer/cord
- Thumb drive
- iPod, MP3 player, Kindle, tablets, etc.
- Adapter for electrical outlets in country where you are traveling
- Speakers for your iPod, MP3 player, etc.
- Chargers (for computer, iPod, Kindle, etc.)

- Video camera
- Lantern and/or flashlight
- MRS/PEMF travel cord (used with an earthing device I always travel with)
- Night guard, if you use one (mouth support for the night grinders and more)
- Passport, credit card, insurance card, calling card
- Binoculars
- Headband (for winter and to protect your ears from the draft on flights)
- Scarves (decorative or for cold weather)
- Extra water (after flying, it's always refreshing to have in your checked-in luggage) when you're feeling tired and dehydrated from flying
- Food (check the list above). Make sure to take your favorite comfort foods and don't forget to take a small container of coconut oil.
- Coffee substitute and/or tea bags
- Stevia
- Wein Products' ozone breath device (helps to oxygenate the air near your body) http://weinproducts.com/frontpage.htm
- Sound machine (for the insomniacs and light sleepers, like me)
- Alarm clock, watch
- Running/exercise clothing (shoes, hat, reflective vest, etc.)
- Heart-rate monitor (for die-hard athletes)
- Hair clip, tweezers, nail clippers
- Spiritual / Altar items (deck of goddess/god/blessings cards and other inspirational material)
- Protein shake ingredients and your Magic Bullet or Nutri-Bullet

How to Best Support Yourself during Travel

- Wear your EMF devices that neutralize harmful electromagnetic frequencies from Bioelectric Shield ([http://www.bio electricshield.com/DrBenson](http://www.bioelectricshield.com/DrBenson)).I am very selective and have researched many companies, and this is my #1 choice.

- Consume eight ounces of water every two hours.

- Move your body to avoid deep vein thrombosis (DVT).Try yoga exercises for the neck, wiggle your toes and stretch your legs out often. (See exercise suggestions from our fitness experts in Chapter 3.)

- Say prayers or mantras to calm your nervous system.

- Read or just enjoy the scenery, it's also a great time to people watch.

- Listen to audio books, which beautifully pass the time away.

- Use essential oils to boost your immunity and your moods, such as Peace and Calming, Lavender and Surrender by Young Living Essential Oils (www.ylwebsite.com/robynbenson/home).

- Use earplugs or a good headset to block out unwanted noise and wear an eye mask at night.

- Wear comfortable clothes and clothes that are protective from EMFs, etc. (See Chapter 10.)

- Diminish your exposure to solar radiation by traveling at night, whenever possible, and taking astaxanthin and the Core 6 Supplements.

- **Drink Plenty of Water**: Keep yourself well-hydrated throughout the flight and all travel. It is best to make sure you are getting adequate water one full week before departure, including a high-water-content diet (lots of fruits and vegetables). This is called *eating your water* and supplies you with high-quality vitamins and minerals. You should drink six to eight glasses of water a day. It is fine to add liquid minerals or sea salt to your water for proper absorption. I am a big fan of Oxylent powdered mineral drink that you can get at your favorite health food store or at Santafesoul.com. Oxylent packets are very easy to carry in your pocket or purse. Reduce caffeinated beverages and high sugar drinks, which can cause dehydration and make you feel loopy.

- **Hydration**: The HCT always knows to hydrate. It's great to add liquid chlorophyll or Aerobic 07 (Chapters 4 and 9), and use your portable structured water unit faithfully for all water, coffee and even alcoholic beverages. I like the device (as mentioned in Chapter 4) by Clayton Nolte sold by the Wellness Enterprise (https://bhe88838.isrefer.com/go/specialoffer/a172/). At the Tesla Tech Extraordinary Technology Conference where I presented, one of the doctors measured the before and after results of exactly what happens to each and every person's energetic field after drinking structured water from this portable device and it was amazing! He used a Gas Discharge Visualization (GDV) camera. The structured water becomes more accessible to our cells, circulation increases and people feel more energized. To see a video, go to http://thewellnessenterprise.com/.

- **Avoid Caffeine and Alcohol**: These two can be very dehydrating, especially while flying, and having one alcoholic beverage in the air is actually the equivalent of drinking two or more, due to the altitude. You should also limit your sugary drink intake. Why? These beverages can send your 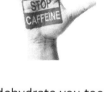 blood sugar on a roller-coaster ride and dehydrate you too, especially when you are traveling at 30,000 feet.

- **Eat Lightly**: Food is harder to digest at high altitudes, so eat lightly during the flight and avoid the high-salt, high-fat foods that the airlines, airports and convenient stores tend to serve.

- **Get Up and Stretch**: Stretching stimulates your circulation—and be sure to dress comfortably. Learn more about stretching in Chapter 3.

- **Expose Yourself to Natural Light**: When you arrive, get your feet on the ground right away and expose yourself to as much natural daylight as you can. Light is the most powerful influence on the timing of your body's internal clock.

- **Consider Melatonin**: You can take .3 to 3 mg at bedtime for two to four nights to significantly reduce jet lag, regardless of the direction of travel. Also, as mentioned above, taking melatonin two to four days before departure or on your way home can make your transition easier.

- **Get 8+ Hours of Sleep**: Always aim for at least eight hours of deep REM sleep per night. Take natural sleep supplements (chapters 5 and 9) and add magnesium for its calming effects, for sore muscles and to help keep your bowels moving. Sleep in complete darkness and electro-sanitize your sleeping space at least one hour before bedtime.

- **Plan Ahead**: Try planning the next day's activities the night before to avoid early morning rushing around and annoying delays.

- **Emergency Protocols**: Same as pre-travel.

- **Health and Nutrition Protocols**: Find local food restaurants and connect with your destination through the story of food, especially when in foreign countries. This is easy to do when eating tapas in Spain, dining in sushi bars in Japan, enjoying outside cafes in Paris or the outdoor food scene in Thailand, where the aromas of spices and oils will whet your appetite from afar. Find places where you actually taste the beauty.

- **Supplements**: Continue with the Core 6 Supplements, and iodine and astaxanthin to protect against radiation. (See Chapter 9.)

- **Motion Sickness**: Wearing a wristband on your P6/Nei-Kuan acupressure point can be very helpful. There are also stickers you can put behind your ears that help to resolve motion sickness. I also recommend a supplement by Health Concerns called Quiet Digestion for all of my patients who are susceptible to motion sickness.

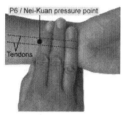 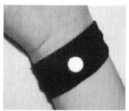 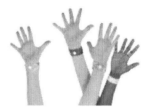

How to effectively electro-sanitize your hotel room

- **Book your hotel room** on the ground floor or first few floors, because the higher you go the further you are disconnected from the earth frequencies.

- **Bring an EMF/Gauss scanner** to assess electro-smog spots in your hotel room.

- **Pack protective sheets** (Earthing Sheets) or at the very least protective EMF protective clothing to sleep in (see Chapter 10).

- **Unplug all unnecessary electronic items** in the bedroom, especially near your head, so there will be less exposure to harmful frequencies in your room.

- If there is **a wireless phone in the room, move it** as far away from the bed as possible or unplug it all together. Do not sleep near any electrical outlets; a distance of at least three feet away is best.

- All clock radios plugged into an outlet are high in EMFs. **Travel with your own portable clock** and disconnect all plugs and clocks in your hotel room.

- More than likely, the room next to yours has all the electric outlets against the wall that is close to where your head is while sleeping. **Consider sleeping with your feet toward the head of the bed** and your head at the end of the bed.

- Fans, air conditioning and heaters are high EMF devices. If you need white noise, **bring your own portable device** and use heating and cooling systems only when absolutely necessary. Research shows it is better to sleep in a room that is around 65 degrees. So get cozy under blankets rather than having the heat on, when possible. Learn more at sleep-foundation.org.

- Of course, you will remember to **drink lots of water**! Hotel air tends to be dry and can be dehydrating.

Protect Yourself during Ground Travel

How many hours a day are you in your car? The average person drives about 12,000 miles per year. There are many ways you can protect yourself from the high EMF levels you are exposed to every time you turn the key and drive anywhere. Grocery stores and shopping malls also contain high levels of electromagnetic pollution. Some of my EHS patients cannot even walk into a shopping mall or a Starbucks, due to the Wi-Fi and other high frequencies found there.

Electronic gadgets in your car, such as a GPS, mean increased EMF exposure as well. The more electrical your car is, the more hazardous it is to your health. I'm sorry, Prius owners. If you drive a hybrid car, have an internal GPS system and your stereo is turned on, you are swimming in a sea of EMF frequencies. If you doubt this for a second, take your gauss measurement device out to your car and check for yourself. Chapter 10 has a complete list of travel solutions that will help mitigate EMF exposure while helping your body stay energized and healthy.

Jet Lag and Post-trip Lethargy

Hydration and a healthy diet are the best antidotes to jet lag and travel fatigue. It also helps to take melatonin two days before and a few days after air travel. Melatonin does not work for everyone. Hydration and a healthy diet allows for a smoother transition for everyone. This is also a time to consume things like green drinks and low-sugar smoothies. Do your best to stay awake and fall asleep at your new bedtime. Also, the MRS/PEMF device that I and many other travelers use has a 24-hour clock that acclimates the body

to the current time zone, thus making it
easier to fall asleep in your new time zone.
(Visit Chapter 9 for more information.)

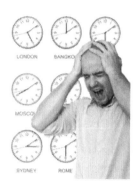

The most common symptoms of jet
lag include:

- Headaches

- Fatigue, irregular sleep patterns,
  insomnia

- Disorientation, grogginess, irritability

- Mild depression

- Constipation or diarrhea

Lemon added to your water will help you to efficiently detoxify
from your travels. Continue to eat high water content fruit and vegetables in order to keep your cells, your brain, and organs functioning well. Remember to get out in the sunshine as much as possible
when you get back, to fortify your moods and energy. Walk barefoot
to re-ground. (For more information see Chapter 9.)

Supplements: Continue on the Core 6 Supplements for at least
a few weeks post travel.

Sleep: Always aim for at least eight hours of sleep.

Planning: If you are a frequent traveler, as you unpack, refill
shampoo containers, replenish your supply of extra batteries, and
refill your supplement containers to make sure you are ready to go
for the next time you travel.

Health Protocols: Resume a healthy lifestyle as usual.

Travel Tips for Special Circumstances

Women traveling alone

I can honestly say, I love to travel in all ways: with friends, family,
groups and alone. I have traveled solo to many states and countries. Several of my best travel experiences have occurred alone,
where I tend to meet more people and fit as much as possible into
every day. I truly love to be on my own schedule! Fortunately, I have
had mostly positive experiences traveling alone because of following the guidelines below.

More than anything, I have learned the importance of self-empowerment and always intending to be grounded and in control. I remember running in the wild with my Masai friends in Kenya, where at any turn a lion or a gazelle could appear. The Masai taught me to always carry my body in a posture that represented power and strength rather than fear and ambivalence. I have never forgotten this sage advice, no matter where I am.

How to be safe and secure

I want you to know about this, HCT, in order to avoid a travel nightmare! HomingPIN is the world's first, truly global lost property **and recovery** system. I love this system and have the sticker on all my valuables (credit card, suitcase, phone, camera, etc.). Protect your bags, keys, cell phone, cameras and more, from loss. To find out more, see http://www.homingpin.com/.

I met Andrew Hopwood, the manager of this company, and was thrilled to find that 2,000 airports now recognize this system. Bravo, and what a great way to travel with more confidence that your lost belongings could be returned with ease. Inadvertently leaving our valuables behind just happens in the rush of travel. However, following the Healthy Conscious Traveler's Blueprint for your individual needs can make a big difference in preventing anything, from getting sick to missing planes and trains to losing your valuables.

- Always travel with your phone everywhere you go, even if you go out for a run.

- Get to know the front desk people or concierge of your hotel. Let them know your destination and that you are going out for a walk, run or hike on your own. Leave a note with friends, coworkers or others to say where you are going.

- Since I have traveled alone a lot, I always believe "I have eyes all around my head." In other words, be incredibly aware of your surroundings at all times. This is especially important if you run alone and are in unfamiliar territory.

- When going on day trips, be prepared with food, identification and money, and know your destination.

- Do not get into unmarked cabs—ever!

- When getting in and out of cars alone in parking lots, talk or pretend you are talking on your phone. Make a lot of noise.

- Notice suspicious people in parking lots, hotel lobbies and deserted streets.

- Clothing can draw attention to you, so make good choices to avoid trouble in any bar or social situation while traveling alone.

- Take a self-defense class in your hometown. Consider taking a karate class or building core strength by taking Kettle Bell or CrossFit classes.

- Do not accept rides from strangers.

- Always be fit throughout your life—no exceptions! It is not only a serious health risk to be carrying an extra 30-plus pounds, but it makes you much less mobile when you need to act or run quickly, or kick an offender where it hurts.

Children traveling alone

If a child of yours has to travel by themselves, here are some tips to make it easier and more stress-free for everyone involved, including you as the parent as well as the airline and flight crew and the person picking up your child at the other end of the journey.

Follow All Health Protocols as Outlined above, and Adjust for Your Child: Yes, it is best for your child to travel when rested, well-hydrated and with a healthy immune system.

Is Your Child Ready? No two children are the same at any given age. Consider the maturity and personality of your child when deciding if they are ready to make a trip alone.

Prepare Your Child for the Trip: Let your child know the details of what to expect, such as how long the wait will be, who will pick them up, etc.

Talk to Your Child Regarding Appropriate Behavior: Your child should know what type of behavior is expected of them. It is essential that they understand they must show courtesy to the flight crew and other passengers. They should also know what to do if there is any inappropriate behavior toward them from other travelers. Of course, no passenger should ever solicit information from them like their full name, their address, their phone number, their destination or any other personal information. Make sure your child knows that they should contact the flight attendants or airline personnel if they encounter any problems.

Know Your Airline's Policies: Make sure to review and understand your airline's policies about unaccompanied children. Pay extra attention to their rules regarding how a child is escorted to connecting flights and what happens if a flight is delayed, diverted or canceled. Each airline's rules are a little different.

Get There Early: Plan to arrive at the airport earlier than normal. This will give you extra time to deal with any last-minute situations and to help your child feel safe.

This Chair Is Just Right! It is important to make sure the seat assigned to your child is convenient and appropriate. When making the reservation and checking in your child at the airport, if possible, try to have your child seated in a row with empty seats on one or both sides of them. Request that your child not be seated in a row with passengers drinking alcohol. If it is allowed, escort your child all the way to their seat on the plane to make sure they are safe and comfortable. This will likely keep you and your child more calm and happy.

Find the Person in Charge: Once on board, you or your child should find the lead flight attendant and/or the flight attendant in charge of the area in which your child will be sitting. Making personal contact will often make for an easier flight for your child and make you feel better.

At the Destination: Whoever is meeting your child at his or her destination should be fully prepped with all the pertinent details of your child's flight. Ask that the pick-up person gets to the airport early and confirms that they have picked up your child. If possible, try to have a back-up person lined up to meet your child, just in case.

Traveling with children

Almost all of you have probably been in this situation: You are just settling into your seat as you prepare to leave on a flight. Down the aisle comes another passenger with one or two children in tow. You think to yourself, "Please don't sit next to me. Not here, not here, please not here." Why do we think this? Because children, as wonderful as they are, can be a nightmare when cooped up in an airplane cabin for hours on end. As parents or grandparents, aunts, uncles, or friends, there are some things you can do to make plane flights more tranquil, comfortable and even enjoyable when traveling with kids.

Shiny and New! You definitely want to bring some favorite toys, games and books with you to keep your child occupied. Consider also getting some new items for the trip. Surprise them with something they have not seen before. This will likely keep their attention for some time and make the plane ride an even more special occasion.

Bend the Rules! Even if you have a rule about your children not watching television, a long plane flight is not the place to enforce it. If there is an appropriate movie or show playing on the airplane's screens, let your child watch it. This can keep them occupied for a long time, which you, and the other passengers around you, will greatly appreciate! Same goes for tablets, phones and so forth. Download a couple of fun game apps or digital copies of their favorite movies. No harm is done, and the novelty of being able to do something normally off-limits will make the trip even more appealing.

Diaper Time! If you are traveling with children using diapers, do yourself a favor and prepare ahead of time for the inevitable in-flight diaper change (or two or three). In your carry-on, have a few diapers ready with a plastic bag inside of each. Once on the plane, stuff a couple of these diapers and your changing mat into the seat back pocket. Like this, you are ready to handle diaper changes without the hassle of accessing the bag in the overhead compartment each time the need arises—and it will!

Travel in Comfort: When traveling with children, keep it simple. Consider having your children travel in their pajamas. They will think it is fun and will be comfortable should they want to nap, plus you will only have to pack an extra set of pajamas or two for the inevitable outfit change (think spills, diaper issues, etc.). Don't forget to pack an extra t-shirt for yourself too, because when kids vomit, spill juice or whatever, they usually (read always) seem to include their parents in the fun.

Look, Don't Touch! As you, along with millions of other people, make your way through airports, shuttles, restaurants and so forth, your kids will want to not only see but touch just about everything they come in contact with. The tactile issue is big for kids, and very natural, but not so sanitary. When traveling with children, always have your favorite anti-bacterial hand cleanser or wipes with you.

Carry-on Sanity: You will thank yourself a thousand times if you limit yourself to one carry-on. Keeping your eye on one or more children in a busy airport can be challenging enough! Don't burden yourself with multiple carry-ons to manage. However, if your child is old enough, let them bring their own carry-on. This way they can bring along their own toys, books and possessions, and have a sense that they are really helping out by taking their own bag, just like mommy and daddy!

Time to Eat! Meals served in flight are famously mediocre, if not downright horrible. There is very little selection (chicken or beef?), and as passengers, we are at the mercy of the flight crew as to when we get to eat. All of this may, or more likely may not, jive with the food needs of your child. Be prepared by always traveling with some of their favorite snacks. If traveling internationally, make sure these snacks don't violate any customs rules. Also, make sure the snacks don't need refrigeration and are hardy enough to withstand the rigors of travel. Saltine crackers and strawberries are probably not a good bet.

Travel for the elderly

BEFORE YOU TRAVEL

- Talk with a travel agent. Many travel agencies specialize in senior travel and can help find the perfect destination for you.

- Research online or buy a guidebook to learn about the language, culture, climate and more of your chosen destination.

- If you are traveling in a wheelchair or with a guide dog, be sure to contact your airline, hotels and tour companies in advance, to make the necessary arrangements.

- Consider purchasing travel insurance and make certain that it covers pre-existing conditions.

- Research the places you will be visiting so you are familiar with the medical facilities available.

- Follow the news to keep up with any changes in the weather, flight cancellations, airline strikes or any type of unrest or natural disaster in your destination country.

PACKING

- Make sure your carry-on has everything you need for your day of travel, such as your Healthy Conscious Traveler's First-Aid Guide (www.robynbenson.com), prescription drugs, a change of clothes, a book, music or anything else you may require.

- If you take prescription medicines, use a pillbox that has the days of the week marked on it and filled up with all the pills you need for each day. While traveling it is easy to get out of your daily routine. Having the pillbox prepared will help keep you on your personal regimen.

- Use only suitcases with wheels. Rolling your luggage through airports and hotels is far easier and more convenient than carrying your bags.

- Pack comfortable, non-binding clothing. This not only makes travel more pleasant, but also lets your blood circulate more easily during long periods of inactivity.

Traveling with a disability

- Make any special arrangements you may require well in advance of your departure. Check in with airports, airlines, hotels and shuttles regarding special dietary requirements, seating arrangements, wheelchair accommodations and other needs.

- Whenever possible, book direct flights. If that is not possible, make sure to allow sufficient time to make your connections.

- If traveling abroad, contact the embassies of the pertinent countries to check on their rules regarding wheelchairs, guide dogs, etc.

Traveling with medication

- If traveling internationally, assure your medications are legal in the country or countries to which you are traveling. To do this, contact the embassy or consulate of those countries.

- Talk with your doctor about what medicines you will need for your trip.

- Ask your doctor to write you a letter stating what medications you are taking, the dosage and that it is only for your own personal use.

- Take the original bottles of your prescription medicines so you can refer to dosage instructions. This may also help when going through customs.

- If you inject your medication, you may want to take your own needles and syringes. If you have to buy them overseas, make sure the packs are sealed and sterile.

The pre-travel doctor visit

- Get a complete check up with your doctor before you leave, especially if you have heart disease, hypertension or any other chronic condition. While you are there, talk to your doctor about any health concerns you have about your trip, including your medication, vaccinations or differences in the cuisine of where you may be traveling. Those with diabetes will need their doctor's advice on how to adjust the timing of their medications when traveling to another time zone.

- Travel can often mean long periods of time sitting in planes, trains, and buses. This has been associated with blood clots, especially if you have poor circulation. Check in with your doctor about this if you have concerns.

Safety first

- Be sure to add your Homing Pin stickers to all your valuables! Visit http://www.homingpin.com/ and enter coupon code HT2015 to receive a 20% Healthy Travel discount.

- Be attentive and look out for unwary travelers. Pickpockets and thieves are everywhere, especially at popular travel destinations and wherever there are a large number of people.

- Instead of a purse or regular wallet, consider using a money belt or a travel wallet with a cord that goes around your neck or is secured to your belt.

- Whenever you put your carry-on down, always place it between your feet and loop the shoulder strap around a chair leg when possible.

Don't leave home without

- Your passport (if traveling abroad) and make copies to have in case you lose the original

- Phone numbers for the US embassy in the countries to which you are traveling

- Contact numbers for your airline

- Phone number of your travel agent (if you used one to arrange your travel)

- Emergency contact numbers of relatives or friends

- Phone numbers for your doctor(s)

- Your prescription medicine

Traveling with pets

If you are an animal lover, chances are you will be traveling with your furry buddy. Here are some basic FAA regulation regarding traveling with pets:

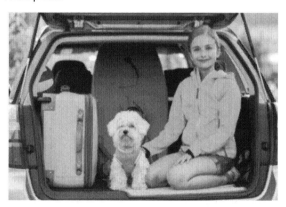

- Your pet container must be small enough to fit underneath the seat without blocking any person's path to the main aisle of the airplane.

- Your pet container must be stowed properly before the last passenger entry door to the airplane is closed in order for the airplane to leave the gate.

- You must follow flight attendant instructions regarding the proper storage of your pet container (http://www.faa.gov/passengers/fly_pets/cabin_pets/).

Also, make sure to follow up on your pet's booster shots and airline pet allergy policies (http://latimesblogs.latimes.com/booster_shots/2010/02/pets-allergies-airplanes.html).

The Humane Society of the United States recommends that you do not transport your pet by air unless absolutely necessary. If your pet must travel in the cargo hold, you can increase the chances of a safe flight for your pet by following these tips.

- **Use direct flights**: You will avoid the mistakes that occur during airline transfers and possible delays in getting your pet off the plane.

- **Always travel on the same flight as your pet**: Ask the airline if you can watch your pet being loaded and unloaded into the cargo hold.

- **When you board the plane, notify the captain and at least one flight attendant that your pet is traveling in the cargo hold**. If traveling during the summer or winter months, choose flights that will accommodate the temperature extremes. Early morning or late evening flights are better in the summer; afternoon flights are better in the winter.

- **Fit your pet with a collar that can't get caught in carrier doors**. Affix two pieces of identification on the collar: a permanent ID with your name and home address and telephone number, and a temporary travel ID with the address and telephone number where you or a contact person can be reached.

- **Affix a travel label to the carrier** with your name, permanent address and telephone number, final destination, and where you or a contact person can be reached as soon as the flight arrives.

- **Make sure that your pet's nails have been clipped** to protect against their hooking in the carrier's door, holes, and other crevices.

- **Do not give your pet tranquilizers** unless they are prescribed by your veterinarian. Make sure your veterinarian understands that the prescription is for air travel.

- **Do not feed your pet for four to six hours prior to air travel.** Small amounts of water can be given before the trip. If possible, put ice cubes in the water tray attached to the inside of your pet's kennel. A full water bowl will only spill and cause discomfort.

- **Try not to fly with your pet during busy travel times**, such as holidays and the summer. Your pet is more likely to undergo rough handling during hectic travel periods..

- **When you arrive at your destination, open the carrier as soon as you are in a safe place and examine your pet**. If anything seems wrong, take your pet to a veterinarian immediately. Get the results of the examination in writing, including the date and time.

For Medical Conditions

See Chapter 9: *Smart solutions for your top health challenges.*

International Travel and Health

See Chapter 9: *Smart solutions for your top health challenges.*

Chapter 9

Smart Solutions for Your Top Health Challenges While Traveling

It's not the years in your life that count, it's the life in your years. ~ Abraham Lincoln

People are dying too long and living too short.
~ Dr. Bruce Bond, D.C.

It's a fact that travel stresses your immune system, adrenals, and nervous system. In addition, many people are now experiencing adverse health effects from a variety of visible and invisible environmental toxins, including the effects from industrialized foods, chemically contaminated water, toxic homes and body care products, not to mention the side effects from pharmaceutical drugs.

In this chapter, you will learn about smart solutions for the most common travel health challenges. This chapter is divided into two sections, with the first addressing the most common travel-related ailments. The second section addresses how to remedy these health issues with natural herbs, foods and drug-free choices.

It is critical that you learn to honor and trust what I like to call your *inner-nature pharmacy*; it is what keeps you breathing, digesting, energized and detoxed 24/7. You may take for granted your 70-plus trillion cells, your brilliant organ systems, hundreds of hormonal pathways, your magnificent brain, immune system and much more, all endlessly working for you. But remember, you have an intelligent body that has an innate ability to prevent and reverse illness if you simply feed it what it actually needs to stay healthy.

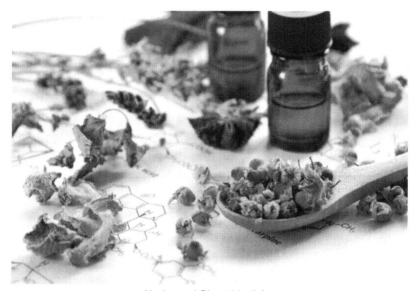

Herbs and Plant Medicine

Did You Know That There Are at Least 50,000 Medicinal Herbs Worldwide?

Years ago, as a young acupuncture student, I learned that there are more than 10,000 herbs in the Chinese medicine pharmacopeia alone. This was evident to me on my three-month trip to three provinces in China, where I studied with renowned doctors of herbology. I was in awe at the endless selection of bones, leaves, berries, nuts and seeds, all used in formulas to heal anything from pain to inflammation and skin disorders.

In the West, we are fortunate to have vitamin and herb stores in just about every town and supermarket and, increasingly, in airports and convenience stores. But my friends in near and faraway places have shown me that there is nothing like picking plants, food, and herbs directly from the local earth, and brewing them as medicinal teas to cure headaches, anxiety, respiratory infections and other ailments.

One of the great benefits of traveling as a health practitioner is that my lifelong desire to learn about medicinal herbs has been satisfied. I have taken herb walks in Africa, Bali, Peru, Bolivia, Haiti, China, Egypt, Sardinia, Mexico and Nicaragua. It is common for the native people of these lands to remind us that Mother Earth provides. Over and over, I heard that most everything you could possibly need for food and medicine is found within 15 miles of your home. I heard this specifically from Q'ero Indians of Peru, Masai of Kenya and the Curanderos of Mexico.

This way of living, by the way, is how most of the world lives. Unfortunately, in the United States we are often led to believe that toxic, synthetic drugs are the only way to treat *most* modalities, from depression to cancer. I can tell you that is absolutely not the case after 23 years of working successfully with patients and confidently treating people with acupuncture, IVs, injections and my own natural pharmacy (all non-prescription). In addition, I encourage all my patients to follow The 8 Pathways, to avoid and prevent sickness. However, I am grateful for the emergency medical system this country provides. It is equally comforting to witness the massive growth of integrative and functional medicine, where doctors help their patients not only to get to the root of their health challenge but to look at all the systems that are involved (thyroid, adrenals, digestion) that have caused the body to break down in the first place. Once this is decided, it is possible to turn most chronic conditions around.

With so many choices for the HCT traveler, it can be confusing choosing which herbs and vitamins to focus on. To solve this issue, I have created a Healthy Conscious Traveler's First-Aid Kit (robyn-benson.com) with emergency essentials for such conditions as:

- Headache
- Constipation

- Diarrhea
- Anxiety
- Jet lag
- Trauma from a fall
- Cuts and burns

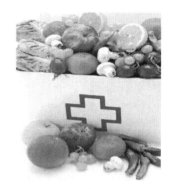

Top products for the healthy conscious traveler's first-aid kit

- Probiotic/enzyme blend (Biotics) or one you do not have to refrigerate, for easy travel
- 85%+ Dark Chocolate (rich in minerals, antioxidants and first aid for a big sugar craving)
- EMFbioshield (EMF protection) http://www.bioelectric-shield.com/DrBenson
- Soap-free shower gel (Nutribiotic)
- Jet-lag homeopathic www.nojetlag.com or visit Jetzone www.antijetlag.com and www.jet-stress.com
- Lavender wipes (calming and sterilizing)
- Arnica topical or tablets (good for pain, bruising and even sleep!)
- Quiet Digestion from Golden Flower (all digestive disorders and even jet lag)
- Gabatrol x 2 (for acute stress, anxiety, heart palpitations)
- Melatonin .3 mg to 3 mg (for sleep), from Natural Health International
- Activated charcoal(detox, binds toxins)
- Barlow's LDM-100 (antimicrobial) (tincture of Lomatium) barlowherbal.com. Use code D79QX1G4C for 10% discount
- Biofreeze - topical (pain reliever)
- Isatis Gold (Health Concerns)

- Emulsified Oregano Oil (Biotics brand excellent for virus, bacterial and fungal infections)

- Grape seed extract (good for parasites, virus, bacteria and fungus)

- Oscillococcinum from Boiron (for first sign of cold or flu)

- Cayenne is excellent to stop bleeding and even for a heart attack

- Turmeric is helpful for acute and chronic inflammation and is a powerful antioxidant

- Coriander oil is an excellent way to help treat any kind of food poisoning, yeast overgrowth, dysentery or diarrhea. It also helps you absorb vitamin D! http://store.activation-products.com/coriander/offer?AFFID=189434

- Triphala (Ayurvedic fiber for constipation) or 500-1000 mg magnesium for constipation

When in doubt, and based on where you travel and your allergy predispositions, pack a general first-aid travel kit that includes: Benadryl, Band-Aids, Aspirin, Neosporin and an Epi-Pen if prescribed to you and **get medical attention immediately when needed**.

Using your intuition is an essential part of being an HCT. Listen within to know if you or a fellow traveler is in danger and needs urgent medical care (Pathway 8).

Bring your attention once again to the Stress, Electrified Times thermometer in Chapter 1. If you want to thrive during your travels, it is best not to leave your home while you are in the Red Zone, depleted and running on empty. If you travel when you are in the Yellow Zone, you have a small reservoir to deal with the unexpected, and it is best to support your adrenals and immune system by following the Healthy Conscious Traveler's blueprint in Chapter 8. My advice is to live the Green Zone lifestyle on a regular basis, so you will be maximizing your body's precious resources.

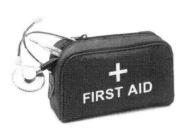

When you travel, your inner pharmacy may need a little boost and extra TLC when any of the following health challenges show up.

Section 1: Common Travel Health Concerns

Allergies

Due to the increasing number of toxins in our environment, more people suffer from allergies today than at any other time in history. While traveling, you may be allergic to your pillow, hotel furniture, detergents, mold, unfamiliar foods and certain pollens without even knowing it.

You are more prone to allergies when your major organ systems are out of balance because of stress, poor eating habits, and being in new environments while traveling; i.e., hotel rooms, new rental cars and beach areas with mold. Your best defense is a healthy immune system. Make sure you are getting enough healthy fats, and increase your antioxidants (vitamins A, C, D3, E, Selenium, Zinc, Glutathione and Quercetin).

My two favorite herbal recommendations for allergies are Histoplex from Biotics Research and Allergena, a homeopathic remedy that is zoned for different pollens throughout the country. I feel strongly that allergy sufferers should always carry Benadryl for the unexpected allergy reaction, since Benadryl can save your life! However, I am not a fan of taking Benadryl for sleep. There are much better choices. Whether you're eating a food that catches you by surprise and your throat swells or you get stung by a jellyfish or you accidentally touch a poisonous plant, please have Benadryl and an Epi-Pen (epinephrine). Never leave home without this, or another type of antihistamine, nearby especially for your children. Check to make sure your current Epi-Pen prescription is up to date. When my son was young, he had a few serious allergic episodes, so even at age 15, he always has an Epi-Pen on hand, just in case.

Do your research and find hotels that cater to HSPs (see Chapter 7) and other people who have a tendency to be more al-lergic to indoor and outdoor environments. I stayed at a Doubletree hotel in San Diego where they put me on the sixth floor, for people who prefer sheets without perfumes. A year ago, I stayed in an L.A. Marriott that has rooms with Ozone air purifiers. It was heaven to stay in such a room. Cheers to Double Tree, Hilton Hotels and a few Marriott Hotels that are listening to their growing clientele who make these requests. I sure do!

Altitude sickness

A small percentage of travelers experience strong altitude effects when arriving in high-altitude destinations (such as Santa Fe, NM, Mount Shasta, CA, Nepal, etc.). Common symptoms include headaches, nausea, dizziness, and fatigue, although individual reactions are highly variable. The medication prescribed to prevent symptoms is acetazolamide (Diamox) taken twice daily, starting 24 hours prior to ascent and continuing for two to three days while at altitude (don't take if allergic to sulfa drugs). As a doctor of Oriental medicine, I prescribe the Core 6 Supplements, liquid chlorophyll, *lots of water*, specific Chinese herbs for moving *qi* (energy) and herbs that build blood. For my anemic patients, I recommend a liquid iron gluconate called Floradix and a sublingual B12/folic acid.

When traveling to Peru and Bolivia, all my local friends are quick to give me coca tea (*mate' de coca*) to counter the effects of high-altitude travel and to help renew my energy. *Mate' de coca* is a natural alternative and can be used in a homeopathic preparation as well. Consider buying this tea ahead of time for your high-altitude travel. This is a must for the adventure traveler.

Atrial fibrillation (AF)

This is a condition where the heart skips a beat or has an irregular heartbeat (arrhythmia) and is more common in people who are over 50 and overweight. AF can be accompanied by dizziness, sweating, and chest pain. Please note that left untreated, this condition could lead to a stroke. Most aircrafts are required by law to have a defibrillator. Please review my top 10 food choices (Chapter 2) and take at least 600 mg/day of magnesium to prevent AF, and stay away from high-sodium soups and processed foods. Magnesium is an essential mineral that plays an important role in heart regulation. Hydration is essential to prevent AF.

Bed bugs

These little nasties are more common than you might think. Just like mosquitos, some people have the right skin, odor and pH that attract bed bugs. People who get hives are more prone to bed bug bites. Your best defense is a healthy immune system. Make sure you are getting enough healthy fats, increase your antioxidants (vitamins A, C, D3, E, Selenium, Glutathione, and Quercetin) and always have Benadryl or a natural antihistamine on hand. I recommend Histoplex from Biotics (Chapter 10). A great remedy to prevent and kills bed bugs is a product called Proof at www.bugproof.com. If you're traveling, spray your luggage before you go, during your trip, and when you return, and you'll be protected for weeks

Bladder infection

Getting a bladder infection while traveling is not fun! You can easily avoid this, like all conditions, with proper hydration, avoiding stress and eating a plant-based diet. If this is caused by sex (especially when it has been a while), then invest in Sylk, an excellent, all-natural lubricant. If you are prone to bladder infections, always carry a bottle of D-mannose or even a product with cranberry and d-mannose. Both cranberry and mannose are excellent for getting rid of infection while building a healthy bladder ecology. Also, I recommend never to leave home without a bottle of oregano oil (included in the Healthy Conscious Traveler's First-Aid Kit). I prefer an emulsified form of oregano oil (ADP by Biotics). This is handy for all types of infections (fungal, viral, bacterial and even parasites).

Blood clot prevention

This can be fatal, so make sure you are hydrated at all times before, during and after travel, and eat *clean*. Be aware that blood clots are more common in women who take the estrogen hormone and in people who have arteriosclerosis, a disorder characterized by a thickening and stiffening of major arteries This can be determined by a blood test and further testing by your doctor. People with this condition often have what is known as thick and sticky blood (a sign of inflammation or a low-grade infection) and is more common in people with high blood pressure and increased levels of C-reactive protein and homocysteine. One of my favorite supplements for thick blood is Nattokinase (see below).

To prevent blood clotting, commit to an exercise program and be sure to eat your inflammatory-reducing diet as outlined in Chapter 2. To refresh your memory, consume berries, dark green vegetables, tart cherries, ginger, turmeric, grass-fed beef and fish that is full of omega-3 fatty acids, B vitamins and iron. Also, after working with hundreds of patients, I know it's important to stay away from most grains and gluten products, which are high-inflammatory foods for many people.

Blood sugar regulation and binge management

Maintaining proper blood sugar levels is your key to healthy moods and body weight and one of the most important ways to age well and to avoid most all diseases. Don't make your vacation an excuse to eat poorly! My top recommendations to manage sugar cravings are cinnamon, PGX (a great supplement that supports blood sugar levels, cholesterol levels and weight loss), chromium polynicotinate (200 mcg) and alpha lipoic acid (600 mg).

Constipation

Gastrointestinal complaints are one of the most common health problems in the U.S. and one of the most common ailments I see in my practice. Why? Because most people do not eat enough daily fiber, especially when on the road. It's not surprising when you travel that your intestinal system gets disrupted even more than usual. To have a positive bowel experience while traveling, increase your fiber by eating a plant-rich diet. Also Triphala is a very inexpensive Ayurvedic herb available in most health food stores and it's a fiber that helps keep your bowels moving. It is not habit forming. Stay away from all the over-the-counter brands because most of them contain nasty chemicals. Proper hydration is also important in preventing constipation and is even more important when taking fiber supplements.

Dehydration

Dehydration is a very serious condition and can be life-threatening. Therefore, it is recommended that all travelers drink plenty of water several days before your trip (at least 64 ounces, or half your body weight in water per day), during your travel, and days after you return. Consider consuming your water through food that naturally has a high water and mineral content such as organic fruits and veggies and coconut water.

It is one thing to drink water, yet what is most important is that you absorb the water you drink into your cells. The best way to ensure this is to add a pinch of sea salt to your drinking water or a package of my favorite vitamin/mineral supplement called Oxylent.

You can prevent many common travel-related illnesses simply by being properly hydrated. I highly recommend the book, *Your Body's Many Cries for Water: You Are Not Sick, You're Just Thirsty—Don't Treat Thirst with Medications!* by F. Batmanghelidj. Truly, almost all diseases and many emergency health crises are rooted in dehydration.

Diabetes

Diabetes is a common disease in which your blood glucose, or sugar levels, are too high. There is Type 1, formerly called insulin-dependent or juvenile diabetes, that some people are born with and Type 2 diabetes, which often happens later in life. If you are Type 1, be sure to always have your medications by your side. Keep yourself hydrated and eat clean organic, non-GMO food as much as possible.

Sugar, flour and refined carbohydrates found in most processed foods play a big part in the development of Type 2 diabetes. The average American consumes 150 pounds of refined sugar per year, so it is not surprising that diabetes is becoming increasingly common and is the root of many other diseases, including heart disease and cancer. To avoid the sugar highs followed by the "sugar blues" during travel, it is best to adhere to your healthy diet.

Diarrhea

The "runs" are common with travel, especially when visiting developing nations. Cinnamon bark and peony make an excellent

Chinese herbal combination (from Golden Flower herbs) that is useful as well. Take four capsules before each meal, beginning three days before your trip and throughout the trip. Also consider coriander, already mentioned above. This is a great alternative to Pepto Bismol with the same effect, and it's a healthier choice for your body. To protect against diarrhea and bacteria in the intestines, take two capsules twice a day of Acidophilus and Bifidus or Saccharomyces Boulardii before meals, beginning on your first day of travel and throughout the trip. I also recommend activated charcoal to bind toxins and to help stop diarrhea. Once again, this is a condition that can be debilitating, even life threatening, as it can cause severe dehydration. Be sure to get medical attention if you cannot get it under control.

Digestion, stomach upset and gas pain

Gasalia from Boiron is probably one of the best homeopathic supplements available to quell uncomfortable gas and bloating. I also like Quiet Digestion from Health Concerns for almost any nausea, or abdominal upsets (and it is even helpful for jet lag.) Do not leave home without it. Stay away from Tums and other over-the-counter gas-reducing products, as they are full of chemicals and won't solve your problem. Also, as much as you want to be adventurous with food, consider the consequences of what you choose to eat and the complications that may arise from ingesting unfamiliar foods.

DVT

The risk of deep vein thrombosis (DVT) is greater in passengers traveling in packed economy class seats, where there is little room to move. It is more likely to happen to people known to have circulatory blood issues. To reduce the risk of DVT, try clenching your calf muscles at regular intervals to stimulate blood circulation and make sure you get up and move about hourly to encourage circulation throughout your body. Don't cross your legs as it cuts off circulation. You can also wiggle your feet and massage your lower legs, knees and ankles. Try wearing support hose/socks when you travel, to lessen the amount of fluid accumulation. My #1 recommendation is www.vitalsox.com.

Also invest in NEO40, or http://www.neogenis.com, (use HTS10 at check out for Healthy Conscious Traveler discount) as this product helps to increase nitric oxide, which is a gas that helps to improve circulation. Make sure you drink plenty of water (at least eight ounces of water per hour of travel) and avoid caffeine and alcoholic drinks, as these can dehydrate the body.

Ears

Similasan Ear Relief and garlic/mullein oil are excellent for ear problems. Also, consider oregano oil (ADP) from Biotics and Isatis gold from Health Concerns for ear infections. If either of these do not get rid of the infection, consult a doctor for treatment to avoid a serious ear drum rupture. Use earplugs to drown out high-pitched noises, and if pressure builds in your ears, pinch your nose shut and swallow while trying to push air through your pinched nostrils.

Edema

The simple solution to prevent unnecessary edema when flying and traveling is to drink nothing but water, avoid all salty and unhealthy foods three days before and during travel, and stick to a healthy diet. If you are prone to edema, please consult with your healthcare practitioner since edema is often a sign of a minor/major imbalance in your body, especially relating to your kidney function, electrolyte levels and your ability to detox efficiently. Edema is often a sign that there is more fluid outside your cells than inside your cells due to these mentioned stressors. Try wearing support hose/socks when you travel to lessen the amount of fluid accumulation. My #1 recommendation is www.vitalsox.com.

Estrogen pollution (EP)

More and more people have too much of the hormone estrogen from plastics, canned drinks, food additives, and more. The best herbs for estrogen dominance are Meta 13c, and calcium d-glucarate, and of course, stay away from the aforementioned culprits and consume the Healthy Conscious Traveler's anti-inflammatory diet as outlined in Chapter 2.

Eyes

Your eyes often need extra tender loving care when traveling. This is due to the dry air in most all indoor-travel choices, from cars to planes. A natural way to treat dry eyes and keep them moist is with BioTears by Biosyntrx or Dry Eye Relief by Similasan. Choose the one that fits better for your exact symptoms. For puffy eyes, consider putting wet chamomile tea bags over both eyes and even cucumber slices, and of course, avoid high-sodium, inflammatory foods.

Eye products with zeaxanthin, lutein and berry extracts such as bilberry and blueberry are excellent for overall eye health. If you suffer from a chronic eye issue and want a natural approach, visit the Ocular Nutrition Society to look for a natural eye care doctor. Always protect your eyes with very high-quality sunglasses when outdoors. Your eyes are especially vulnerable to sun damage at higher altitudes. I always travel with eye antibiotic/steroid drops just in case of contracting conjunctivitis or any type of eye infection. This has come in handy more than once while traveling with my children. When I spoke to a pilot recently, he mentioned how toxic solar flares can be to our eyes, and his remedy is to drop lower in the sky to protect himself and the passengers. And of course, close the window shade near your seat.

Fatigue

Follow the Healthy Conscious Traveler's blueprint as outlined in Chapter 8 to significantly reduce fatigue associated with last-minute running around and stressful packing. Realize *effortless* travel is possible with proper preparation. With hundreds of causes for fatigue, your best bet with travel is to take a good quality B complex vitamin and eat food that is alive and promotes energy production in your cells. Fatigue while traveling is more common with a diet full of empty calories and processed grains such as donuts, bagels, and muffins. Consider eating fruits high in natural sugars such as bananas, strawberries and blueberries and, as always, *stay hydrated*. A big part of fatigue while traveling is dehydration and chronic adrenal fatigue (discussed in Chapter 6), which is very common, living in today's very stressful world.

Fear of flying

In my research, it appears that 30 to 40% of people experience some level of stress and anxiety about flying. Please consider any or a combination of the herbs I list under *Stress* in this section. William Langewiesche, one of the most articulate people on the subject of flying, says that on a typical US airline, your chances of dying on a flight are somewhere around one in 13 million. Many therapies can help with the fear of flying, from hypnotherapy to repatterning and the popular EFT method of tapping (see Chapter 10).

In his blog, Nick Ortner, creator and executive producer of the hit documentary film, *The Tapping Solution*, says, "Follow the tapping trail and consider this therapy for all your fears, because deep anxieties and trauma often affect multiple parts of people's lives. Ask yourself what's at the root of your fear of flying—a feeling of being unsafe? Not being in control? Not trusting the people who fly and maintain the plane? Once you get your answer, take some time to consider how these issues are affecting other parts of your life, whether it's your sleep or your relationships. Then use tapping to work through those issues as well." Ortner recommends tapping before, during and after you fly.(1) To get a copy of his free eBook, *Tapping Your Way to Health, Happiness and Abundance*, visit www.The TappingSolution.com.

Fibromyalgia (FM)

This autoimmune disease manifests with chronic pain, often in the shoulders, back and buttocks. Most people with this condition have trouble sleeping and some also experience spasms and bouts of severe depression. Travel can be particularly aggravating to the FM patient. I always recommend the trifecta: water, minerals and a water-rich diet free of any chemicals and preservatives. Increase your magnesium levels and all other herbal anti-inflammatory supplements (EFAs, turmeric and green tea). From my own clinical experience, this condition, among many of these mentioned in this chapter, is reversible. Find a qualified doctor who can help you get to the root of this condition.

High blood pressure (HBP)

Hydration is one of the best ways to manage healthy blood

pressure. If you take prescription medicine for HBP, please continue to take it as scheduled. Travel is not the time to reduce or change your prescriptions. Also, manage your stress to prevent high blood pressure spikes while traveling. If you have HBP, travel is an even more important time to consider a very healthy diet low in sugar, bad fats and alcohol consumption. My favorite remedies for high blood pressure are hawthorn berry, 600 mg of magnesium, at least 200 mg of CoQ10 and a great nitric oxide product called NEO40, created by Dr. Nathan Bryan. Listen to his great interview on www.healthy travelerssummit.com to find out about this effective product. I also recommend a sublingual B-12/folic acid supplement to all my patients with high blood pressure. These two vitamins also help manage your ideal blood pressure. Jeff Primack, in his book *Conquering Any Disease*, says that eating six stalks of celery a day will dilate your arteries and lower your blood pressure.

Infections

There are several types of infections, including bacterial, viral, fungal, and parasitic infections. For most all infections, use isatis gold, oregano oil, LDM-100 (see below), vitamins A, D and thieves oil (http://www.ylwebsite.com/RobynBenson/home).When traveling, especially internationally, I recommend having an extra antibiotic on hand for when the above do not work. Ask your doctor for a Z-pak (azithromycin) or another antibiotic in case you contract an acute infection while away. By following the Healthy Conscious Traveler's blueprint in Chapter 8, you can prevent this from happening in the first place!

Other great choices that I offer my patients are intravenous therapies, such as vitamin C, or the popular Myers cocktail, which are both loaded with vitamin C and other immune-stimulating vitamins/minerals that will boost your immune system. (See IV therapies listed in Chapter 10.)

Jet lag

1. Drink plenty of water. Keep yourself well-hydrated before and throughout the flight.

2. Avoid caffeine, alcohol and sugary drinks. These beverages can send your blood sugar on a roller coaster ride.

3. Food is harder to digest at high altitudes, so eat lightly during the flight and avoid the high-salt, high-fat entrees the airlines and airports serve.

4. Dress comfortably and get up and stretch now and then to stimulate your circulation. Learn more about stretching in Chapter 3.

5. When you arrive at your destination, expose yourself to as much natural daylight as you can. Light is the most powerful influence on the timing of your body's internal clock. You can buy travel lights for this purpose on Amazon.

6. Consider melatonin. You can take .3 to 3 mg of melatonin sublingually or swallow a capsule or tablet at bedtime for two nights before long-distance travel to significantly reduce jet lag, regardless of the direction of travel. Take melatonin around the time you desire to sleep at your new destination to get your circadian rhythms on track with your new time zone. My favorite melatonin product is Herbatonin .3 mg and Herbatonin Pro 3mg by Natural Health International.

7. Invest in a program called Stop Jet Lag. It is possible to arrive at your destination feeling fresh, regardless of the time zone. Stop Jet Lag offers an easy-to-follow, individualized plan for your specific itinerary. It's based on a natural approach that safely and effectively resets your body clock by correctly timing your intake of food, drink, sleep, bright light and optional melatonin supplements. There's no guesswork, and mobile alerts make it even easier. Thousands of travelers have successfully eliminated jet lag with this plan.(2)

8. Consider taking Jet Zone (arnica, gelsemium, nux vomica, etc.). Follow instructions on the box for best results. Some of my patients swear by this product.

Low oxygen

At cruising altitude, airline cabins have air pressure and oxygen levels that are lower than normal. Blood oxygen saturation during commercial flights can be 5% to 10% lower than normal. If you're in good health, your body can compensate. But if you have a lung condition, such as chronic obstructive pulmonary disease (COPD) or cardiovascular disease, you may need supplemental oxygen even if you don't normally use it. Ask your physician for advice several weeks before your flight.

If you need oxygen, call your airline to find out its policies and costs. Airlines generally require advance notice, and the FAA doesn't allow passengers to bring their own oxygen supply on commercial aircraft. Most airlines require a letter from your doctor confirming your need for supplemental oxygen, along with the required oxygen flow rate. You'll need a copy for every flight segment.

Malaria

Malaria is a mosquito-borne infectious disease that afflicts people in many areas of the world. To avoid this serious, sometimes fatal disease, I recommend that anyone traveling to potential malaria zones take preventative medicine to avoid being stricken by malaria. The prescription drug Malarone (atovaquone/proguanil) has proven most effective without strong side effects. *Artemisia* (wormwood) is a good herbal option. I also like to use citrus oils to (lemon and orange) keep the mosquitos away.

Mold exposure

I believe this a major health challenge with travel and more than people realize. If you go to a beach area, it is very common to find mold on ceilings in the bathroom, in the air conditioner, in vents and in corners. Yet mold can be found in all climates. I have a nose for mold. Mold exposure is debilitating to many people around the globe. I have left hotel rooms many times after discovering mold. I get a headache, my nose immediately gets congested, and brain fog sets in. I vividly remember taking my son to Ireland when he was only six months old. He had bad case of eczema and was already immuno-compromised before we left on this trip. After an hour of being in our hotel room, he immediately became swollen all over his face and ankles. He had trouble breathing and I started looking around the room and found mold in many different places. Best strategy if this happens to you while traveling is first to get another room or hotel, and follow the recommendations under the allergy section in terms of supplement and essential oil support. Mold sensitivities are often indicative of needing some detoxification support, and a sign to clean up your diet, digestion, and your overall gut health.

Nausea and vomiting

In Chinese medicine, both nausea and vomiting are signs that the *qi* (energy) is moving in the wrong direction. Both of these are rather common with travel, with various stomach flus and certainly with any type of food poisoning. Altitude changes, turbulence and poor food choices can also stir up an unhappy digestive system. Quiet Digestion (Golden Flower Herbs) and Curing Pills (made by several Chinese herbal companies) are excellent choices.

Nux vomica is a well-known homeopathic medicine for nausea and digestive upsets. Often it is best to avoid solid foods with this condition and instead choose chicken broth and other easy-to-digest foods. I always travel with low-sodium miso soup in a convenient package for these moments. It's also nice to have handy when I am craving a warm beverage. Be sure to pack your wrist bands, mentioned in Chapter 8, if nausea and motion sickness are common for you. Also make sure you get enough B6 to avoid travel related nausea.

Neck pain

Neck pain and stiffness is probably one of the chief health complaints among frequent travelers. Finally there is a well-made pillow, a neck support system, that works when you are a passenger in a plane, train, bus and in cars. I met the inventors of this system at the annual Travel Goods Show. This is the best sleep system I have seen for the Healthy Conscious Traveler. Go Sleep has released a truly effective, upright sleep system designed to allow today's busy traveler a restful sleep "*on the GO.*" It includes several features such as a pillow carrying case that can be used for neck or back support. The premium sleep mask sits away from the face and allows eye movement. An adjustable elastic cord with toggles secures to the seat or adjustable headrest, comfortably supporting the head in place. To find out more: www.gosleepusa.net.

Restahead is another excellent and reputable neck travel aid. All you do is bend it, put it behind your neck, and relax into a comfortable position for sleep without falling into your neighbor's lap. I use mine not only for travel but also when I meditate. It is lightweight and great for travel.

Neck support in hotels

For relief of neck pain while in any other bed but your own, I highly recommend the Tempur-Pedic travel pillow. Every hotel has a different type and quality of pillow, so either bring a pillow from home or invest in a great travel pillow that is comfortable for your neck. An injured neck can set you up for miserable travel, so be sure to pack what you find best for your needs. The travel pillows sold in airports are certainly helpful for sleeping on the plane, but some are pure junk and are full of toxic plastics and fabrics, so beware.

Pain

A great acronym for P-A-I-N is Pay Attention to Internal Nurturing. With our fast-paced lives, we often move and do so much that we neglect ourselves and our inner alarms that tell us to slow down and listen to what may be the source of the pain. When we continue to ignore or suppress pain, it often intensifies until it is too late to make the necessary changes to erase the pain naturally.

There is a worldwide epidemic of people suffering with pain. The National Institutes of Health reports that 100 million Americans are affected by pain.(3) There are endless causes of pain, including inflammation, genetics, food sensitivities and overuse injuries. Common treatment is over-the-counter aspirin and ibuprofen for general inflammation and narcotics such as codeine and morphine for more severe pain. Your best approach to manage pain while traveling is to combine traditional pain management with complementary therapies. You can now find massage therapists and mini-spas in many airports and in just about any city to which you travel.

If you prefer a complementary approach (chiropractic, acupuncture and naturopathy) to your pain or travel ailment, contact the concierge at your hotel or do an Internet search of your destination before you travel. Many of these doctors are also trained in trigger point injection therapy, B12 injections, and IV therapies for a variety of health issues, from fatigue to infection. Arnica salves and biofreeze are perfect topicals to take with you on all trips for muscular pain and bruising.

Parasites

Oregano oil, black walnut and clove oil, grapefruit seed extract and artemisinin are all effective natural remedies for parasites. Visit http://www.ylwebsite.com/RobynBenson/singles. I am partial to artemisinin, since I was fortunate enough to spend some time with a physician who was a leading researcher in the natural prevention and treatment of malaria in Kenya. I travel with both oregano oil and clove oil that I put on the bottom of my feet before sleep. This is great for your immune system and to even get rid of parasites. Because the oregano oil does not smell good, I always put a light sock on. I also recommend LDM-100 and Mycocyde and Clarkia 100 and several other herbs from barlowherbal.com.

Radiation exposure (discussed in chapter 1)

One of the best ways to protect yourself against radiation is to take iodine daily (6.25 mg). The only exception to this is if you have an autoimmune thyroid problem. Increasing your intake of greens (including cilantro, and nori) is an excellent choice for your continued protection against radiation exposure. Astaxanthin is also recommended. Always remember that having adequate blood levels of vitamin D (at least above 50) is necessary for overall health. The beauty of cilantro (also known as coriander) is that it helps you absorb vitamins A and K, which are necessary for vitamin D synthesis.

Sciatica

This can be a very painful, sometimes debilitating condition and is not fun to have while traveling! Long-term sitting can aggravate sciatica, a set of symptoms caused by irritation of nerve roots in the lumbar spine. Commonly, there is pain felt in the lower back/buttock region, down the back of the leg (usually on one side or the other, not both) and often past the knee and down into the foot. Besides pain, sciatica can also cause numbness, tingling, muscular weakness and inability to control the leg. The best treatment for sciatica is acupuncture and chiropractic care. Often an injection can be effective. Many people choose cortisone shots, but you might consider alternative choices that I offer to my patients, such as trigger point injections, Prolozone Prolotherapy shots, and Platelet Rich Plasma injections. I offer all of these excellent choices to my patients but not cortisone. The injection therapies that I offer help to heal the origin of the pain rather than treat a temporary band-aid effect.

Sinus

Sinus ailments are common for the traveler, since you often put yourself in a contained environment with very little oxygen, which can become a breeding ground for viruses, bacteria, funguses and other critters. If you are prone to sinus problems, bring your Neti pot with you. You can buy it at any pharmacy or health food store and most come with everything you need. I also recommend adding ten drops of liquid iodine to your Neti pot. Plan to do your nasal rinse at least twice a day before you travel and while you are away. Most sinus issues can easily be prevented with proper diet, by avoiding your known food sensitivities, getting proper rest and getting out in the fresh air on a regular basis.

The two most important supplements for sinuses are a good antihistamine and oregano oil. I prefer Histoplex from Biotics Research or Aller Plus from Progena. Biotics Research also has a great oregano product called A.D.P. This is one of the best all-around natural antibiotics. Take three tablets, three times a day in addition to the Core 6.

The **Core 6** (as seen in Chapter 8) are: 1) a quality multivitamin/mineral supplement; 2) magnesium 600 mg; 3) probiotics; 4) extra vitamin C (4 g/day) and zinc 30 mg; 5) vitamin D (at least 2,000 - 5,000 IU); and 6) B-complex.

Skin reactions

From poison oak and poison ivy to hives, the best topical remedy might be the gel from the aloe plant or aloe gel products to reduce inflammation or calamine lotion to deal with the itch and help to dry up the blisters. Also, Barlow Herbal Specialties' Golden Salve may help to soothe your skin and is always great to have in your smart traveler's kit. Go to the nearest hospital if you have any difficulty breathing. For other skin conditions, consider homeopathic creams such as chamomile, Bach Flower Rescue Remedy cream, and if possible, take a bath with a box of baking soda that alkalinizes and soothes your skin. This folk remedy has been around for hundreds of years and is known to ameliorate the itching and burning associated with skin problems. Internally, you can take ACS Silver 100.

Sleep apnea

This sleep disorder interrupts a person's breathing while sleeping, sometimes hundreds of times a night, depriving the brain and the rest of the body of oxygen. Travel with your CPAP machine or other device, and also consider working with a health care professional who can help you get to cause of your apnea. Obesity, a sedentary lifestyle, and a lack of certain minerals and amino acids can be common causes of sleep apnea.

I was thrilled to find out about this easy to travel with CPAP machine for people with sleep apnea. While you may go on vacation, sleep apnea never does, so it stands to reason that sleep apnea sufferers should never leave home without their CPAP. The small and lightweight Transcend CPAP is an alternative to lugging around a full-size CPAP unit. The Transcend Travel CPAP allows travelers to easily bring the therapy they need to maintain the benefits of healthy sleep. Find them here at www.minicpap.com.

Stress

Remember to breathe and to bring awareness to your breath is what is most important when it comes to feeling stressed or being in a stressful situation. In addition, stress tamers are found in supplements such as De-Stress from Biotics, Gaba and Pure Life Gabatrol and Free and Easy Wanderer from Golden Flower (good for hormonal balance too).You can also travel with another calming amino acid called theanine. Holy Basil and Ashwagandha help to tame the stress hormone cortisol. I also recommend herbal calming teas and Calms Forte rescue remedy cream and liquid. I suggest these excellent remedies to my chronically stressed patients to restore their adrenal glands, which can often get seriously weakened with regular stress.

Throat pain

In your Smart Traveler's First-Aid Kit, be sure to have a supply of Thayer's Slippery Elm Sugar-Free lozenges for throat pain. Slippery elm is also good for stomach issues and is a natural antibiotic. I recommend a good echinacea-based throat spray to help with immune support and to reduce a sore throat. I am also a big fan of gargling with sea salt to moisturize the inflamed throat tissue.

Varicose veins

This malady is very common, especially in people 50 and older. Varicose veins are veins that have become enlarged and raised above the surface of the skin. This occurs when the valves in the veins that prevent blood from flowing backwards stop working properly. This allows blood to pool in the veins, causing them to enlarge. Any vein can become varicose, but it is most commonly found in the legs and feet, because standing and walking increases pressure in the veins of the lower extremities. I recommend investing in quality support hose or socks (www.vitalsox.com) to avoid any complications.

Vertigo

A person with vertigo often feels as though things around them are moving, even though they are stationary. Vertigo is usually caused by an inner ear problem, though other issues can cause it as well. Vertigo is more than just dizziness. It is a persistent sense of spinning, swaying, tilting, and such. Symptoms can last from several minutes to several days or longer and may include nausea, vomiting, blurred vision, lightheadedness, earache, and a loss of balance. For quick relief, press acupressure point P6 on your wrist (refer to Chapter 8) or find an acupuncturist. I also recommend you find a chiropractor to adjust your neck to restore optimal alignment. Too often, because of funky sleep positions on airplanes or while driving for extended hours, the cervical and thoracic vertebrae get out of alignment.

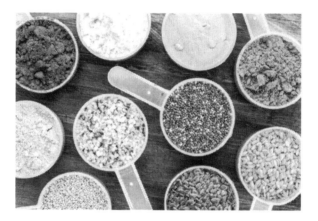

Section 2: Top Herbs, Supplements and Super Foods for Healthy Travel

Cold and flu prevention plan

FOUNDATIONAL SUPPLEMENTS

Multivitamins and Minerals. In today's world, everyone needs a basic multivitamin and mineral supplement. The research is overwhelming on this point. As our soil has become more and more depleted over time, most of the food we eat is mineral deficient. Find a quality multivitamin with antioxidants and minerals. Personally, I like our Self-care Revolution products that you can find at www.santafesoul.com. I have tested thousands of patients for vitamin and nutrient deficiencies and found that people feel better once they correct these deficiencies. Of course, vitamins are secondary to a wholesome diet, but sadly, in my experience, I am seeing that many people do not make the food choices that support vitality and well-being.

Vitamin D should be considered among the primary non-pharmacological agents to protect against low-radiation damage and even radiation-induced cancer. What is your vitamin D3 level? It is best to have your level above 50 ng/ml. This can be determined by a simple blood test from your health care practitioner. Most people are severely deficient and I see this daily in my practice. Vitamin D deficiency can cause a host of problems including depression, thyroid problems, muscle pains, and immune deficiency. Spend as long as it takes, supplementing vitamin D (1,000-10,000 IU/day) and getting outdoors without sunscreen for at least 20 minutes with 40% of your body exposed to the sun to optimize your vitamin D levels. Please understand that it can take months, even years, to achieve the correct level. Many studies show an association between low levels of vitamin D and respiratory tract infections. Adequate levels of vitamin D will help boost your immune system so you have stronger protection against many ailments.

A study published in *The American Journal of Clinical Nutrition* found that only 10% of school-age children who took vitamin D got the flu, compared with 18% who took a placebo.(5) For most children and adults 2,000 international units (IU) daily is acceptable. Increase to 5,000 IU/day during peak flu months (January through March). This is higher than the dose I typically recommend, which is 1,000 to 2,000 IU, but these higher doses of vitamin D are safe. Children and infants can take 1,000 IU daily, then increase to 2,000 IU during peak flu months, though for infants, check with a pediatrician about increasing the dose. I recommend that all people who travel on a regular basis take a minimum of 5,000 IU/day, regardless of sun exposure, due to radiation and other hazards of traveling.

Zinc is also chronically low in most people. I test all my patients with a zinc saturation test by Biotics Research or Standard Process. Find a practitioner in your area who uses these products and offers the zinc test. Zinc is integral in the making of more than 200 enzymatic processes. The body needs zinc in order to produce white blood cells along with selenium and hydrochloric acid (one of the most important digestive enzymes to break down protein). It is also essential for a high-functioning immune system and it helps with tissue healing. As a D.O.M, I've tested hundreds of my patients

over the years, and about 90% are zinc deficient; thus I highly recommend 30 to 60 mg a day.

Vitamin C. I suggest you take 4,000 mg of vitamin C per day.
Vitamin C aids your body in producing collagen, strengthens tissue
and muscles while it boosts your immune system, provides anti-inflammatory support and further protects against viruses and bacteria.

Resveratrol. 200 mg from red grapes boosts your energy production and protects your cells. Resveratrol helps regulate glucose
levels, thus helping with weight management. It also protects
healthy cells from damage caused by exposures to things like ultraviolet (UV) rays and helps to slow down degenerative conditions.

Beta-glucan is an immune modulator. That is to say, it regu-
lates the immune system as opposed to stimulating it. It can activate but never over-stimulates (see http://www.cancertutor.
com/beta-glucan/).

Probiotic. Find a quality probiotic that does not have to be
refrigerated while traveling. I love our brand at www.jointheself-
carerevolution.com/shop. It is critical to take one to three weeks
before travel to build up a healthy gut and immune ecology.

Essential Fatty Acids and Fish Oils (EPA/DHA). Great for reducing
inflammation, depression, and pain. Great for heart and joint health
too. It's also essential for cell wall health of every cell in your body!

Other essential vitamins and herbal products for safe and energetic travel

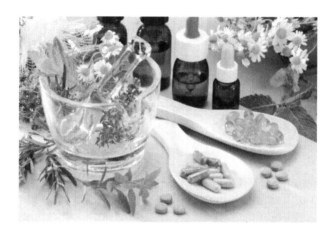

At Santa Fe Soul Center for Optimal Health, we are big fans of **Bulletproof Products** by my friend Dave Asprey. I personally know the quality of these products and travel smart and regularly with all of the ones listed below. I also recommend them to all of my global travelers. Whether you travel to give a presentation or for pleasure, don't you always want to be at peak performance? To learn what Dave Asprey (a professional bio-hacker and the author of *The Bulletproof Diet*) has to say about bio-hacking and upgrading your travel, visit www.healthytravelerssummit.com.

If you still occasionally miss "energy drinks," then try **Unfair Advantage**, which will give you a quick and lasting burst of energy without the crash. By powering up the mitochondrial power plants deep inside your cells, you'll give your brain and body a powerful boost that leaves you standing when all your friends are slumping in their chairs. All in an "ampoule" the size of a pen cap that you can take with you anywhere. It actually tastes good too! http://www.gop jn.com/t/TEFNSUdGQUVGSUpHRkFFRERLR0Y.

Bulletproof Brain Octane Oil. This product is the top choice for reaching peak brain performance all day. For many travelers, you NEED peak brain power as you travel across time zones, and Brain Octane Oil is able to offer maximum cognitive function, converting into energy faster than other fats or oils. This product is 18 times stronger than coconut oil. Brain Octane delivers much-needed ketones to fuel a starved brain that can no longer efficiently metabolize glucose for energy. What I also love is that it brings candida into balance, preventing it from introducing 120+ known toxins into your bloodstream. For travel purposes, it makes meals "bulletproof," optimizing the health benefits, and is flavorless and easy to add to your diet. Mix into any smoothie, soup, sushi, coffee or most recipes for more intense mental activity. Best of all, it is easy to travel with because no refrigeration is required and it's liquid at room temperature. http://www.gopjn.com/t/TEFNSUdGQUVGSUpHRkFFRERLR0Y.

Collagen Protein (CP). If you've looked at the labels on conventional protein powders then you already know that all protein is *not* created equal. Most proteins are damaged during harsh processing and add insult to injury with harmful artificial sweeteners, colorings and flavorings that rob you of peak performance. That's why Bulletproof Collagen uses pure 100% grass-fed collagen powder (the same rare nutrient found naturally in bone broth) that builds lean muscle mass *plus* gives you added benefits unique to collagen, like deeper sleep and even better skin! I add a tablespoon of CP to all my morning travel smoothies. I also keep CP with me in my daypack to have on hand for a low blood-sugar moment or when I have an aches after a workout.

GABAwave. Travel often means *jet lag*. Yet you don't have to "just sleep it off." By boosting levels of the Gaba neurotransmitter found naturally in your brain, GABAwave relaxes your mind to help you focus, fight stress *and* get to sleep faster than ever, even in a strange bed in a different time zone. Better yet, a single dose stays active in your body for up to 36 hours, so you only need to take it a few times a week to get the full benefits. You can even start your day with GABAwave to keep the stress beasties away and to be even more resilient with the ups and downs of daily life. GABAwave may not be the best tasting stuff, but it works (https://www.upgraded self.com/bulletproof-gabawave).

Glutathione. Your body *naturally* makes the best cold, illness and hangover-killer known to science. In fact, this amazing "antidote"–Glutathione–is the most powerful antioxidant in your body, protecting you from toxins, infections and pathogens, heavy metals, inflammation and more. Unfortunately, your liver often doesn't make *enough* Glutathione on its own to maximize your performance. And that's where Bulletproof Glutathione Force comes in, to give you a convenient, highly absorbable dose of Glutathione anytime you need it. Be sure to always include this when you pack your Healthy Conscious Traveler's First-Aid Kit. You can also take NAC (listed below), which is a precursor to glutathione production.

Here is a convenient code to place your Healthy Conscious Traveler's Bulletproof order and to get the latest special: https://www .ugradedself.com/products/bulletproof-upgraded-glutathione-force.

Other excellent travel supplements

Arnica. This is a very popular homeopathic ointment or pill that is widely used for pain, bruising and to heal injuries. I always like to have this available in my travel first-aid kit for the unexpected trauma or injury.

Artemisinin. I am a fan of artemisinin, a natural remedy for parasites, and was fortunate to spend some time with a doctor who was a leading medical researcher in the natural prevention and treatment of malaria in Kenya.

Astaxanthin. A seafood component extracted from algae has some protective effects against oxidative impairment and DNA damage induced by various forms of radiation. The research is sound.(5) Common benefits from astaxanthin use include protection against radiation damage when flying in an airplane and a 4 mg dose can also help prevent sunburn. Astaxanthin can be pricey but worth it.

Bach Flower Remedies. Rescue Remedy, Rescue Cream and Rescue Sleep Bach Remedies are effective in addressing life's stressors: sleeplessness, PTSD, acute trauma, as well as for peaceful transitions and to foster proactive rather than reactive emotions. Do an online search to find a practitioner well-versed in plant remedies in your local area.

Biofreeze is a menthol-smelling, green, gooey, topical ointment used for all sprains, strains and muscular pain too. It is not recommended on open wounds. This is recommended for your first-aid kit.

Chlorophyll has been found to help prevent cancer and is helpful for altitude sickness. It boasts high levels of vitamins A, C and E, has strong antioxidant capacity and helps reduce inflammation. Chlorophyll is a powerful source of readily available magnesium, which helps to make the blood more alkaline. This is good for people who are constantly stressed and tend to sustain high levels of acid in their body. Chlorophyll can help reduce acidity, which fosters a healthier body all around.

Cinnamon is a medicinal spice that has been used in health care for centuries. In its powder form, cinnamon can be conveniently taken to reduce high blood sugar levels evidenced with type 2 diabetes. It can also aid with digestion as well as help treat diarrhea and even fight the common cold. Additionally, cinnamon can help lower cholesterol and boosts cognitive function.

Coconut Oil. This is one of the most health-promoting of all plant-based fats. I recommend that all travelers pack a small container of coconut oil for your skin to use after a shower, to add a healthy glow to your face. It's a way to satisfy your palate when you need a good saturated fat in your diet, which is actually every single day! Hawaiians call coconut water *noelani*, which means "dew from the heavens."

Coconut Water. Second to water, this is one of the best beverages because it is rich in vitamins and minerals. Please note, take your time to find the best quality. Your number one choice is to drink it right out of the coconut. Next best is to buy coconut water in an eco-container where no preservatives or extra sugar are added. Many tropical cultures prize coconut water above all other beverages because of its re-hydrating and health renewing properties.

CoQ10. This oil-soluble, natural antioxidant, synthesized by the body, is required for the production of adenosine triphosphate (ATP), which helps our bodies generate energy on the cellular level. It is one of the most important antioxidants known to the human body. We all produce CoQ10, but the levels decrease with age. Without supplementation, it is difficult to keep your cells' CoQ10 levels adequate. I recommend 100 to 200 mg/day. Find it in fatty fish, beef, poultry and peanuts, one of the heartiest plant sources of CoQ10.

Digestive Enzymes. Many people are not digesting foods properly, which leads to health issues, including obesity, memory problems, blood sugar imbalances, depression and bloating. Why? Because most of us have impaired digestion as a result of making unhealthy food choices over many years, including eating GMO foods known to affect gut integrity. This limits our body's ability to absorb all the nutrients in an optimal way. The best food sources of naturally occurring digestive enzymes are papain, found in the papaya fruit, and bromelain, found in pineapple. Bromelain has been linked to decreasing pain and swelling in various forms of arthritis and even muscular pain.

Hydrochloric Acid (HCL) is another extremely important enzyme that is critical for proper digestion of proteins. It is necessary for the production of white blood cells and restores healthy pH balance in the gut. Perhaps most important is that HCL helps to kill parasites and other pathogens before they can wreck havoc in your body. Sadly, many people are taking antacids, which is the second most prescribed drug after the statins and antacids, which block this acid that is immune protective.

In addition to digesting and absorbing your food, your gut is where you manufacture many of your good mood hormones, such as serotonin and dopamine. Your gut is also the core of your overall immunity, so it is essential that you break down your food for optimal absorption. We often need a little boost from digestive enzymes supplements, especially as we age and when we have stress-filled lives.

ATP (Adenosine Triphosphate) is the fuel in your body that is produced in the mitochondria of your cells. When you are chronically fatigued, sick, or stressed, your ATP production is often low. Chronic diseases are typically a result of long-term decreased ATP production. Four important vitamins that support healthy energy (ATP) production are B2 (riboflavin) and B3 (niacin) as well as the active form of B3, NADH. NEO40, mentioned already a few times here, is also a great choice for energy production.

Ginkgo. This is known for improving blood flow throughout the body, particularly to the nervous system and brain. It is also known for its antioxidant properties and is considered one of the most valuable memory supplements.

Glutathione (mentioned above; learn more here). This is a critical antioxidant found in every cell of your body. A great source of glutathione is mushroom herbs, such as cordyceps, which grows in high-altitude places like Bhutan. They promote the production of glutathione and are loaded with excellent immune and stress relief properties. They are used in metabolic and biochemical reactions, such as DNA synthesis and repair, protein synthesis, prostaglandin synthesis, amino acid transport, and enzyme activation. Thus, every system in the body can be affected by the state of the glutathione system, especially the immune system, the nervous system, the gastrointestinal system, and the lungs. The best way to get Glutathione is via IV, however this can be costly. In addition to Bulletproof Glutathione Force, I also recommend an excellent liposomal Glutathione that actually tastes good, called Tri Forty from Researched Nutritionals. You can also buy a precursor to Glutathione supplement such as NAC (see below).

Grapefruit Seed Extract. With a multitude of benefits, grapefruit seed extract can address chronic issues, such as sinusitis, candida and acne, to name just a few. This medicinal extract aids in the alkalizing of the body, and helps with gingivitis, bleeding gums and even thrush.

Iodine. HCT, as I've already mentioned, this is super important. You need to protect yourself from increased exposure to radiation while traveling (especially air travel). Pilots and airline crews should consider daily use of iodine. Iodine is also recommended for stimulating the thyroid and fights fatigue, depression, weight gain, fibrocystic breast disease, and even food poisoning. Additionally, it assists with other glandular imbalances and helps eliminate viruses, fungi, and bacteria.

Start with a very low dose (6.25 mg), and consult with your physician. Also, enrich your reserves by eating iodine-rich kelp and other sea vegetables. Sinus sufferers, add liquid iodine (20 drops) to your neti pot. I also recommend a Biotics Research product called Liquid Iodine Forte. Women, add this liquid directly on your breast to resolve cysts and reduce breast pain.

Isatis Gold. This Chinese herbal supplement is exceptionally effective in combating viral and bacterial infections and is especially useful during the cold and flu season. I never leave home without this great supplement or oregano oil.

L-Carnitine. This amino acid transports fatty acids into cells for energy, removes lactic acid, reduces fat, and increases muscle mass, thus helping you to experience less fatigue. Take at least 1500 mg twice per day.

L-Glutamine. This supports the immune function, the nervous system and is considered brain and gut food. I prescribe it regularly for my patients with a leaky gut. Some people use glutamine for digestive system conditions, such as stomach ulcers, ulcerative colitis and Crohn's disease. It is also used for depression, moodiness, irritability, anxiety, insomnia and enhancing exercise performance.

LDM-100. I am a big fan of the late Max Barlow's products from barlowherbal.com, especially LDM-100, which is a broad-spectrum plant antibiotic, virostatic, bacteriostatic, fungicidal that helps fight influenza, colds, respiratory and urinary infections, staph and strep infections, difficult viral infections, polio, Epstein Barr Infections, fungus infection, skin infection, warts, etc.). American biochemist Ernst T. Krebs called it one of the most important antibiotic herbs known to man. Twenty percent of people do get a harmless rash from this product, but it will go away in three to four days. Use code D79QX1G4C on website to get a 10% discount.

Maca. I am a big fan of Maca and use it regularly, personally and in my practice. It is easy to add to your HCT kit. Maca is an adaptogen and this means it helps you control stress, keeps your adrenal glands healthy and enhances a sense of well-being. Studies have shown that maca improves strength and endurance and is essential for exercise enthusiasts. Other studies have found that maca curbs depression and boosts libido in people on antidepressants.(6)

Magnesium deficiency is very common and can lead to muscle pain, headaches, constipation, palpitations, fatigue and insomnia. Magnesium is essential for no less than 200 processes in the body. The best food sources of magnesium are green, leafy vegetables such as spinach and cacao. Small amounts of dark chocolate will help maintain healthy magnesium levels. If you decide that you need to supplement magnesium, the ionic form is best, as it is easily assimilated into the bloodstream and reduces the likelihood of loose stools.

Milk Thistle. The things we eat and drink are often not safe, due to herbicides and fungicides in the soil that then run off into the water supply, as well as animals being pumped full of drugs through injection and their food. Milk thistle helps deal with all these toxins, principally through its ability to protect and repair the liver.

Myers Cocktail. This popular IV cocktail consists of intravenous magnesium, calcium, B vitamins, and vitamin C. John Myers, a physician from Baltimore, Maryland, pioneered this course of intravenous vitamins and minerals as part of the overall treatment for various medical problems, for the common cold and asthma, to offer a boost to energy and the immune system, and for pre- and post-athletic events. This is the most popular IV I offer to my patients. Many of my clients never get on a plane without getting their Myers first!

N-Acetylcysteine (NAC). This antioxidant helps prevent the flu and reduces the severity of symptoms if infection occurs. It is excellent for the lungs and is useful for liver detoxification. Dosage: adults and children age thirteen and older should take 1,000 mg daily. Children ages 6 to 12 can take 500 mg daily. At the first sign of flu symptoms, increase to 4,000 mg daily for adults and 1,500 mg daily for children and continue until symptoms subside. NAC is a precursor to glutathione (GSH), which is one of the most important antioxidants for immune and cellular health. I give NAC to all my patients to increase their glutathione levels and find it is cheaper for people who cannot afford intravenous GSH. I strongly recommend NAC to all travelers who are vulnerable to lung infections, especially asthmatics, and for added protection against radiation exposure.

Nattokinase. Derived from a Japanese fermented soybean, Nattokinase is helpful to people afflicted by blood clots, as it is a blood thinner. This is useful to take if you have a predisposition to blood clots and known inflammation, as evidenced by a high SED rate and C-reactive protein. Many people take this, instead of an aspirin, every day with positive results.

NEO40. I am always searching for the best overall supplements that truly make a difference in people's lives.NEO40 is one of those supplements. I was fortunate to interview the creator of NEO40 (Dr. Nathan Bryan) in the www.healthytravelerssummit.com. Be sure to listen and learn how NEO40 Daily naturally replenishes your nitric oxide levels for healthy circulation, blood pressure, and overall arterial health. It can also improve stamina. Help restore and replenish your body's nitric oxide levels with this patented NEO40 Daily formula. Find them here at www.neogenis.com. Use this check out code: HTS10.

Oceans Alive Pure Phytoplankton. I am always looking for products and supplements that stand above a lot of the junk on the market. Oceans Alive is one that I stand by 100%, and it is offered by my super-conscious friend, Ian Clark. Oceans Alive is a plant-based premium super food and the source of all marine based nutrition. To learn more about this mineral-rich marine algae, visit http://oceansalive.com/genetic-selection/?AFFID=189434. To hear my interview with Ian, you can visit www.jointheselfcarerevolution.com.

Oregano Oil. Oregano is one of the most comprehensive medicinal oils. It is anti-bacterial, anti-viral, anti-fungal, anti-inflammatory, anti-parasitic, anti-allergenic and an antioxidant. In addition, this amazing oil addresses any skin condition or irritation. It also helps regulate menstrual cycles and aids digestion by activating digestive juices. Oregano oil is a treasured tool in my Healthy Conscious Traveler's First-Aid Kit and is the most common herbal formula I prescribe from my herbal pharmacy each year. I usually prescribe it in an emulsified form that comes in a tablet. However, I also like the liquid form. Some brave souls drink it directly in water. I prefer to recommend that people put it on the bottom of their feet, near KI Gushing Spring from Chapter 1.Just two drops at night and for children too, can help fight infections.

Oxylent. From a leading worldwide and award-winning supplement company, and founder Lisa Lent, this premium quality 5-in-1 multivitamin formula with vitamins, minerals, antioxidants, amino acids, and electrolytes comes all in one, refreshing drink. Just add water and enjoy the fizzy flavor. It tastes great.

Ozone Therapy. I can't emphasize enough how important this therapy is for getting rid of acute and chronic infections and to help restore injured knees, shoulders, ankles, hips, and other areas of your body. Visit www.robynbenson.com for more information.

PGX. This acts as an appetite suppressant and also balances blood sugar levels, helps with cholesterol and provides proper levels of fiber. I give this to all of my patients who appear to be headed for Type II diabetes. PGX is awesome for combatting sugar cravings too. I thank my friend Dr. John Gray for recommending this supplement in 2008 to a sold-out audience in Santa Fe, New Mexico. Since then, PGX by Natural Factors has been one of my most popular supplements.

Polyphenol Antioxidants. These are phytochemical-bearing foods, found in green tea and most berries, green apples, red apples, broccoli, parsley, cabbage and celery. Increase your intake of all the above for healthier eyes, ears, nose and overall immune support.

Prebiotics and Probiotics. Most health food stores offer these in an array of choices. Beneficial bacteria used in the fermentation process are naturally found in a healthy gut. These microbes modulate the immune system, break down toxins and carcinogens, create micronutrients, prevent pathogenic bacteria from taking up residence and help defend the body against oxidative stress. They also prevent the proliferation of bad bacteria that can lead to inflammatory gut issues and intestinal permeability. Visit www.jointheselfcarerevolution.com/shop.

Protrauma (Progena). Helps reduce muscular pain, inflammation and any nerve pain too.

Quiet Digestion, Health Concerns or Golden Flower. These treat gastric distress, including abdominal pain, sudden and violent cramping, nausea, vomiting, diarrhea, regurgitation, gastric hyperactivity, abdominal distension, poor appetite, intestinal gas, motion sickness, hangover and jet lag—a perfect combination of Chinese herbs that should be a part of your self-care kit.

Reishi and Turkey Tail Medicinal Mushrooms. These mushrooms are effective for liver and immune health and have been known to be effective in cancer elimination and prevention. For more on the medicinal nature of mushrooms, please Google Paul Stamets or Bioneers.org.

Ribose moves sugar into the cells and allows mitochondria to recycle ATP, thereby restoring energy. Excellent for your regular exercise program and for preventing lactic acid buildup in muscles. It also keeps your heart healthy. At 5 g, one to three times a day, people notice improvements in their mood, mental sharpness, memory and ability to focus.

Simalason Ear Drops. Ear Relief drops help clear water trapped in the ear. The homeopathic ingredients stimulate the body's natural ability to soothe the ear and decrease the ear's sensitivity to external factors, such as water, cold, and drafts. They also, reduce the clogged sensation in the ear and return it to a water-free, comfortable condition (http://www.similasanusa.com/ear-relief-homeopathic-ear-drops).

Spirulina is ranked by AARP as the #1 super food for extending your lifespan. The U.N. has identified it as a primary ingredient in the fight against malnutrition worldwide. It is one of nature's near-perfect foods. Spirulina is similar to sea vegetables such as dulse, kelp, nori, kombu, arame and wakame, and is a great source of mineral. Spirulina can reverse the negative effects of radiation.(7)

Triphala. This is a great supplement to have with you at all times as it aids digestion, inflammation and circulation and is rich in antioxidants as well as having antibacterial and antiviral properties. Triphala is a tridoshic, Ayurvedic herb that balances the entire alimentary canal. It is said to be the compost in which beneficial microorganisms can thrive so it should be taken along with probiotics to improve their effectiveness. Most of my patients can prevent constipation simply by taking two tablets of Triphala before bedtime.

Turmeric. The ingredient that gives curry its distinctive yellow-golden color is also known as "the golden spice of life" and has been used in Indian cuisine for thousands of years. Curcumin, the active ingredient in turmeric, has cancer-fighting properties and is used for all inflammatory conditions. A recent study found that curcumin can actually repair DNA that has been damaged by radiation.

Although the aisles of health food stores and major chains are stocked with supplements promising to quell your ills, I stand by those mentioned in this chapter and have prescribed them for years in my practice.

In addition to traveling with herbs and supplements recommended for *The Healthy Conscious Traveler's First-Aid Kit*, it is always prudent to seek medical attention when needed. Contact <u>santafesoul.com</u> if you have further questions.

Chapter 10

Travel Resources: Books, Products and Smart Technology

An investment in knowledge always pays the best interest.
~ Benjamin Franklin

I did then what I knew how to do. Now that I know better,
I do better. ~ Maya Angelou

Imagine what your life would be like if your 70 trillion cells were working optimally every day. You would most certainly experience a sense of clarity, consistent energy levels, optimal metabolic function, ample detoxification and a strong feeling of vibrancy and vitality that no "energy drink" or cup of coffee can provide.

You would not even have to worry about getting sick or contracting a disease. This may sound like optimistic thinking to you, but it is definitely the right mindset for the HCT.

I have never missed a day of work in 23 years, nor have I had to cancel a trip due to illness. I don't mean to boast, but I simply want to make it clear that I do practice what I preach. I want to share with you the pearls of my career so that you, too, will remain healthy and continue to thrive as you travel regularly, adventurously and wildly!

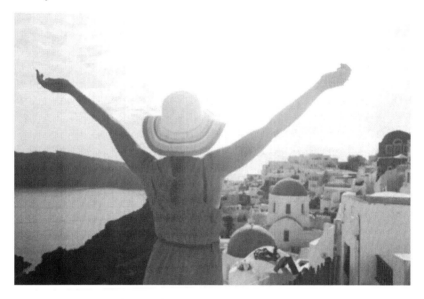

First and foremost, follow The 8 Pathways to Smart and Effortless Travel. This is the key to maintaining your optimum health at all times and especially while traveling.

1. Be your own best health care provider (Chief CEO of your daily health).
2. Reconnect to the earth.
3. Eat real food from natural sources.
4. Drink lots of healthy, potable water in glass and/or BPA-free plastic.
5. Stay active.
6. Optimize sleep.
7. Stay conscious and travel with intention and stress resiliency.
8. Connect regularly to your higher self through mindful techniques.

In this chapter you will review some self-help tools and health resources for your healthy traveling needs. I can tell you I have direct experience with most every resource listed here (see Bibliography) and therefore want you to have easy access to my top choices. This chapter is divided into five sections:

1. Blogs and Health Experts

2. Educational Films and Books

3. Smart Travel Technology

4. Electro-sanitizing Protocols

5. Travel and Health Tips

These resources were extensively researched, and I have personally benefited from them while both traveling and at home. You will find reviews on outstanding educational films, books that cover the adverse effects of electro-smog (negative electromagnetic frequency), advice on wholesome nutrition versus industrialized foods and suggestions for ways to reconnect with the earth.

In the extraordinary technology section, you will find Items like functional clothing to protect pregnant women and children from radiation. This clothing also protects women and men's reproductive areas, which are most susceptible to radiation and negative electromagnetic frequencies, especially while riding motorcycles and on international flights. In addition, you will learn about the Pulsed Electromagnetic Field Radiation (PEMF) mat, probe and pillow system, which mimics the electromagnetic pulsation and frequency of the earth that naturally synchronizes the function of your cells to Mother Earth. You will also learn about self-help tools and tips to electro-sanitize your home, automobile, work environment, and hotel room.

A brief summary will be provided for each resource to save you time and energy with your research. These are, by far, the most credible and reputable sources. Enjoy your self-empowering journey through this educational resource chapter, knowing there is a better way for you to live in this toxic, electrified and most challenging world.

I have discovered, learned and implemented the following recommendations from more than two decades of traveling and professional practice. These are the ways that I have personally been able to sustain optimal health. I am thrilled to be able to share these gems of knowledge with you.

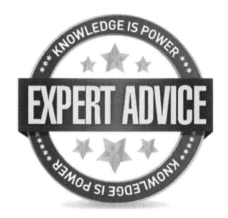

Section 1: Blogs and Health Experts

My favorite health blogs, podcasts and
health experts

Dr. Sara Gottfried, Pedram Shojai

Bestselling author Sara Gottfried, M.D. joins Pedram Shojai O.M.D., founder of Well.org to explore healthy solutions from East to West (http://healthbridgeshow.com).

Dave Asprey

The bestselling author of The Bulletproof Diet talks about how to supercharge your body and upgrade your brain. Be Bulletproof! You can listen to my interview with Dave Asprey here: https://www.bulletproofexec.com, Episode #194 with Dr. Robyn Benson.

JJ Virgin

This acclaimed nutrition and fitness expert and bestselling author has a great program for weight loss and fitness (http://jjvirgin.com).

Nalini Chilkov

Combining her diverse training in Traditional Oriental Medicine, Modern Biomedicine and Cell Biology, Dr. Chilkov primarily serves patients with cancer and complex, chronic illnesses alongside her Optimal Health and Wellness practice (http://nalinichilkov.com).

David "Avocado" Wolfe

The rock star of super foods, this bestselling author has led the environmental charge for radiant health through a positive mental attitude, eco-community building, living spring water, and delicious organic foods and herbs (http://www.davidwolfe.com).

Mind, Body, Green

This informative website is on a mission to "revitalize the way people eat, move and live." Offering tips, tools and ideas to make your life better and to inspire you to keep doing the awesome things that you're already doing, this site is good for your health (http://www.mindbodygreen.com).

Joseph Mercola, M.D.

This bestselling author has a fantastic website and newsletter offering the most up-to-date natural health information and resources. He's also dedicated to exposing misleading information from corporate, government and mass media hype about what is good for your health (http://www.mercola.com).

Rowen Rowen, M.D.

Known as "The Father of Medical Freedom," Dr. Rowen pioneered the nation's first law protecting alternative medicine in 1990, in Alaska (http://www.docrowen.com).

Garry Gordon, M.D.

An internationally recognized expert on chelation therapy, Dr. Gordon is now working to establish standards for the proper use of oral and intravenous chelation therapy as an adjunct therapy for all diseases (http://www.gordonresearch.com).

Frank Shallenberger, M.D.

The Nevada Center of Alternative and Anti-Aging Medicine is a unique, state of the art, full-service medical clinic, with individualized treatment programs for all patients with any medical conditions (http://www.antiagingmedicine.com).

Mark Hyman M.D.

This bestselling author is tackling the root causes of chronic disease by harnessing the power of Functional Medicine to transform health care (http://drhyman.com).

John Cote

The creator and host of Healthcare Elsewhere, a medical tourism show and podcast featuring interviews with doctors, health care experts and patients around the world who travel for Medical Tourism (healthcareelsewhere.com).

Be Well Buzz

This great website strives to "cut through the noise of natural health and wellness" by offering transformative information encompassing wellness within the mind, body and spirit. Their mission is to awaken people to their personal power to achieve transformation (http://www.bewellbuzz.com).

Jonathan Landsman

Founder of a wonderful website full of podcasts, videos and articles devoted to alternative and integrative medicine, he's also host of the Natural News Talk Hour – a free, weekly health show (http://www.naturalhealth365.com).

Environmental Working Group

This nonprofit works hard to empower people to live healthier lives in a healthier environment with breakthrough research and education (http://www.ewg.org).

Bruce Fife

A great source for reliable information on the benefits of all things coconut, from oil and water to palm oil and related topics (http://www.coconutresearchcenter.org).

Section 2: Educational Films and Books

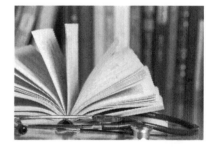

Top book resources

Dirty Electricity by Samuel Milham, M.D. tells the story of Dr. Milham's early years and education and describes his discovery of the link between electromagnetic field exposure and most 20th-century diseases, including cancer, cardiovascular disease, diabetes and even suicide. He alerts people to the dangers of electromagnetic fields and discloses solutions and ways to coexist with the incredible technologies we enjoy today (Electromagnetichealth.org).

Zapped by Ann Louise Gittleman is an empowering guide to living safely with the gadgets we can't seem to live without. Her work is based on the latest scientific data, case studies and information gleaned from her years of clinical practice. This is a groundbreaking guide and master plan that offers strategies as well as super foods and supplements that help minimize the damaging effects of electro-pollution (Areyouzapped.com).

Earthing by Clint Ober, Stephen Sinatra, M.D. and Martin Zucker tells the amazing story of how Ober, a retired cable TV executive, suffered a nearly fatal disease in 1993 and consequently became aware of the benefits of "Earthing." In this book, he describes how our disconnect from the earth has contributed to inflammation, pain, fatigue, stress and poor sleep. He discovered that by grounding yourself by sitting, standing or walking barefoot on the earth or by sleeping on special sheets and pads connected to a metal rod stuck into the ground, you can harness the anti-inflammatory, sleep-boosting and energizing benefits of the natural frequencies of Mother Earth. With some of the open-minded experts in the fields of medicine, physiology and biophysics, he inspired a series of research projects that demonstrated the healing powers of the planet's surface. He also created sleep systems and other devices that help restore our connection to the earth (www.earthing.com/?Click=45538).

To measure electomagnetic pollution in your environment and to find more earthing information, visit my video www.jointheselfcarerevolution.com/deep-healing-frequencies/.

Jet Smart by Diana Fairechild offers great tips and strategies for coping with air travel, based on Fairechild's 21-year career as an airline industry insider. Her career was cut short when she was medically grounded as a result of injuries she received from exposure to unregulated pesticide spraying in aircraft cabins. Her best-selling book *Jet Smart*, published in 1992, exposed the health hazards of flying and played a part in forcing the government to mandate changes in airline policies (lifeinkorea.com/cgi-bin/shopping/book.cfm?ISBN=bb711).

China Study by Dr. Colin Campbell details the connection between nutrition and heart disease, diabetes and cancer. This book is based on a 20-year study conducted by the Chinese Academy of Preventive Medicine, with Cornell University and the University of Oxford. The study was conducted in 65 counties in China and concluded that counties with a high consumption of animal-based foods were more likely to have higher death rates from Western diseases than counties where residents consumed more plant foods. The report also examines the source of nutritional confusion produced by powerful lobbies, government entities, and opportunistic scientists (TheChinaStudy.com).

Your Body's Many Cries for Water by Dr. Fereydoon Batmanghelidj introduces a new paradigm for preventing and treating many degenerative diseases. This highly acclaimed self-help book reveals that chronic dehydration is the root cause of illnesses such as asthma, allergies, hypertension and excess body weight, as well as emotional problems, including depression. He reveals the amazing healing values of natural, simple water. Batmanghelidj presents information that is technically detailed yet easily understood. His viewpoint is based on extensive research as well as personal experience with his patients (WaterCure.com).

Healing Is Voltage by Jerry Tennant, M.D. tells the story of how Dr. Tennant, faced with a serious viral infection in his brain and spleen, discovered a new paradigm in healing. Conventional medicine offered no options for his treatment, and so he began studying cellular biology and eventually created a technology to measure the voltage in each of the organs and also how to correct it. In this book, he explains why body voltage might drop low enough to allow you to get sick. To hear an interview with Dr. Tennant visit www.healthytravelerssummit.com.

Brain Power: Improve Your Mind as You Age by Michael Gelb presents practical, evidence-based wisdom to help you improve your memory. He offers, in clear and accessible terms, practical things that you can do, or stop doing, to continue to improve brain function every year of your life. You'll learn new skills to increase memory, intelligence, creativity, and concentration (MichaelGelb.com).

Healing Traditions, Alternative Medicine and the Health Professions by Bonnie Blair O'Connor explores the importance of culture and belief as organizing principles when one is deciding who to see and what modalities to use when seeking medical treatment. O'Connor is Assistant Professor of Community and Preventive Medicine at the Medical College of Pennsylvania in Philadelphia. In this work, she identifies ways to integrate alternative and orthodox strategies to ensure the best possible care for patients (upenn.edu/pennpress/book/1423.html).

The Geography of Bliss: One Grump's Search for the Happiest Places in the World by Eric Werner is a travel book, but according to Werner "not a typical one." He was a foreign correspondent for National Public Radio for many years, covering catastrophes both natural and man-made. In this book, he travels to some of the happiest places using, as he states, the "science of happiness." His goal was to find out what he could learn from some of the world's most "contented places." His philosophy and humor create an entertaining travel memoir (ericweinerbooks.com).

The Highly Sensitive Person, How to Thrive when the World Overwhelms You by Elaine N. Aron, Ph.D. covers every aspect of the Highly Sensitive Person's (HSP's) life. Aron, who has a doctoral degree in clinical psychology, not only helps to confirm that this sensitivity exists in one out of five people, but also sees it as a gift and points out that the HSP processes everything around them much more than the ordinary person. Because of their ability to reflect, elaborate and make associations, they are able to develop keen intuition, which represents a survival strategy possessed by only a minority of our species.

The Field: The Quest for the Secret Force of the Universe by Lynne McTaggart is a highly readable, groundbreaking classic that reveals the radical new paradigm that the human mind and body are constantly interacting with an interconnected universe. During her research, McTaggart was initially tutored by some 75 quantum physicists, and she presents a layman's view of quantum physics and its metaphysical implications, which is a radical departure from the Newtonian vision of our separateness.

Abundance, The Future Is Better than You Think by Peter Diamandis and Steven Kotler is considered to be an antidote to today's pessimism. Diamandis and Kotler's exhaustive research and extensive interviews with top scientists, innovators and captains of industry demonstrate that abundance for all is within our reach.

Also, inside this book you will find a detailed reference section with graphs, charts and graphics that display the source data supporting the authors' conclusions.

The Charge, Activating the 10 Human Drives That Make You Feel Alive by Brendon Burchard is an inspiring guide that illuminates the path for strategically and intelligently activating the 10 human drives that can put more life into our lives. These drives are critical to your success and happiness, and activating them on a consistent basis will change your life. Burchard has devised what he calls the true "activators," which are a series of powerful yet simple actions you can take to find their charge, share their voice and make a greater difference in the world around you.

The Bulletproof Diet by Dave Asprey offers a blueprint for the right type and amount of food to eat as well as when to eat it and how to cook it. Based on high amounts of healthy fats, moderate amounts of high-quality protein and tons of organic vegetables eaten at the right time, the diet results in unbelievable levels of energy and weight loss.

The Hormone Cure by Sara Gottfried offers powerful tools to reclaim balance and sleep, feel focused and energized, lose weight and more.

Healthcare Elsewhere by John Cote explores how to educate people globally about opportunities that exist for them to travel and receive world class health care at affordable prices.

Top film resources

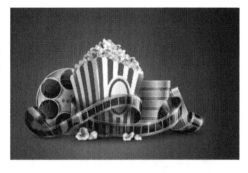

Origins by Pedram Shojai, an ambitious documentary, reveals the simple life that defined our species nearly 200,000 years ago, at the dawning of human exis- tence. This film asserts that the key to our present sur- vival and potential to thrive on this planet lies in understanding the early beginnings of man. *Origins* maintains that the forces that pres- ently compromise our ability to flourish can be overcome by our actual ability to provoke profound and positive change.

Thrive, What in the World Will It Take? by Foster Gamble is a controversial documentary that addresses some of the critical challenges impacting our society today. Featuring interviews with leading progressives, including Amy Goodman, Deepak Chopra, Paul Hawken, Edgar Mitchell and John Robbin, this film examines the nature of the human condition and our ability to prosper (www.thrivemovement.com/the_movie).

Hungry for Change, by James Colquhoun and Laurentine Bosch is an inspiring film that features leading experts in nutrition and natural medicine. It exposes shocking secrets that the diet and food industry have concealed and deceptive tactics that "keep you coming back for more." Learn how you can boost your energy levels, keep excess weight at bay and transform your health through wholesome food (Hungryforchange.tv).

Fed Up by Stephanie Soechtig, a documentary film produced in 2014, focuses on the cause of obesity in the U.S. It presents evidence that the large quantities of sugar and mostly hidden sugars found in processed foods are at the root of the problem. It points out that the sugar industry, with its unlimited lobbying funds, is responsible for this epidemic. This has stymied the attempts to provide a healthier diet for children by parents, schools and states, as well as in Congress (fedupmovie.com/).

Food Inc. by Robert Kenner, Elise Pearlstein and Kim Roberts explores where the food we purchase at the grocery store really comes from, and what it means for the health of our future generations. By exposing the comfortable relationships between business and government, director Robert Kenner gradually shines light on the dark underbelly of the American food industry (Moviefone.com).

Fat, Sick and Nearly Dead by Joe Cross focuses on two men whose bodies have been trashed by steroids, obesity and illness. This documentary chronicles the rigorous healing path, including a two-month diet of fruits and vegetables, that both men traveled in a bid to rescue their health (http://www.hulu.com/watch/289122).

Full Signal, The Hidden Cost of Cell Phones by Talal Jabari explores the effects of our widespread dependence on wireless technology including cell phones, Wi-Fi and satellites. Wireless technology has been dubbed "the world's largest biological experiment ever" by one of the experts featured in this documentary. Through a series of interviews with scientists, health professionals and affected individuals, as well as extensive reviews of the evidence, *Full Signal* makes a compelling case for the need to examine more carefully the effects of wireless technology on our species. Check: http://www.jointheselfcarerevolution.com/deep-healing-frequencies/.

Addicted to Plastic focuses on the worldwide production and environmental effects of plastic. The narrator takes a two-year trip around the world to give us a better understanding of the life cycle of plastic (Topdocumentaryfilms.com).

Forks Over Knives by Lee Fulkerson examines the idea that most of the diseases that afflict us can be controlled and even reversed by eating a diet free of processed and animal-based foods (forksoverknives.com).

Burzynski, the Movie is a highly acclaimed documentary that has won international awards. It tells the true story of Dr. Stanislaw Burzynski, a pioneer in cancer research, known worldwide for discovering antineoplastons, a group of naturally-occurring peptides and amino acid derivatives that act as molecular switches to turn off cancer cells without destroying normal cells. He founded the Burzynski Clinic in Dallas, Texas, to work with cancer patients for whom traditional allopathic cancer treatments have failed. You can watch this impressive documentary on YouTube at: http://burzynskimovie.com/).

Vitality by Pedram Shojai, O.M.D., takes a long, hard look at our broken medical system, a system that uses a mechanistic model of pill-popping, replaceable body parts and the promise of quick fixes that simply mask symptoms. Dr. Shojai's *Vitality* instead presents a practical way for our bodies to flourish through lifestyle habits we can easily adopt. This film directs us to a health-enhancing model that ensures our ability to live life fully and thrive (well.org/vitality).

Bought, The Hidden Story behind Vaccines, Big Pharma and Your Food by Jeff Hays and Bobby Sheehan exposes what is really behind the present expansion of the vaccine program and our dependence on pharmaceuticals and industrialized food. This documentary peels back the layers to reveal how these industries have joined forces as one "super villain." In the film, Hays says that opiates, statins and a blizzard of psychotropic medications do more damage than good. The film explores how our entire healthcare system, from education to practice, has been bought, with stories that reveal corruption, greed, and a shocking lack of conscience from Wall Street (boughtmovie.com/free-viewing/?AFFID=197969).

Unleaded by Shereen Noon, featuring Dr. Roy Heilbron and Angelique Hart exposes an attempt to hide a 10-year, $31 million study conducted by the National Institutes of Health (NIH) on the effects of chelation therapy on heart disease and diabetes. This study involved more than 1,700 patients, and although it was designed to be a definitive study, it was not published by the *Journal of the American Medical Association* (JAMA) until five months later and was ignored by mainstream media. This documentary takes a look at the role heavy metals play in human disease and what chelation therapy can do for heart disease, diabetes and many other diseases by removing metals and toxins from our bodies (epigenetics healthblog.com/tag/unleaded).

Genetic Roulette: The Gamble of Our Lives by Jeffrey M. Smith, a documentary that was produced by the Institute for Responsible Technology, includes interviews with medical doctors, educators, nutritionists, veterinarians and scientists from many different fields. It discusses the relationship of the dramatic increase of food allergies, asthma, autism and other digestive and autoimmune problems as a result of the introduction of genetically modified organisms (GMOs) into the marketplace. In this film, scientists present convincing evidence that the consumption of GMOs causes an array of human health problems (vimeo.com/90061444).

Moldy by David Asprey: Bulletproof Media, 2015.

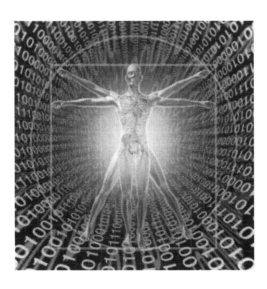

Section 3: Extraordinary Technology and Hygiene

The power of magnetic resonance stimulation (MRS), also known as pulsed electromagnetic frequency technology (PEMF)

One of the best health investments you can *ever* make in your lifetime is to purchase a MRS/PEMF system. These systems range in cost from $2,000 to $5,000, and the PEMF 100 is $26,000, but you cannot put a price too high on a device that has been proven to be one of the best technologies available to combat electromagnetic pollution. As we learned in Chapter 2, the earth's frequency is vital for all life to thrive on a cellular level. The iMRS, or Omnium 1, is a benevolent wellness pulsed electromagnetic frequency device manufactured in Germany that mimics the earth's frequencies, thereby using the power of nature to affect cellular health in only eight minutes.

One of the best aspects of a bioenergetic medicine technology like MRS/PEMF is that you can benefit from it for the rest of your life! That's cheap, for "health insurance."

The MRS/PEMF technology takes under-functioning cells and renews their health. In other words, after a very short session, from 8 to 24 minutes, more oxygen is delivered to each of your cells, and there is faster nutrient exchange and more efficient detoxification. This technology is excellent for alleviating pain, reducing inflammation and inducing deep REM sleep! The iMRS also turns on growth factors, increases stem cell growth and is one of the best devices I know for treating jet lag, as it restores your cells to the right voltage and to the healthy earth frequencies of your current location and time.

Dr. Mehmet Oz highlighted this device as a "cell smart" technology, and supports the idea that we all need this device for healthy living in these electrified times.(1) I want to add here that I am grateful to author John Gray for introducing me to this amazing technology in 2008. He spoke at a sold-out event for our non-profit and told the crowd that this was the best technology that he had come across in his 30-year career in the diet, health and fitness field.

I am a more confident and a much healthier traveler when I bring my iMRS mat along on all domestic and international trips. To date, I have taken my iMRS to 17 countries, and I do not leave home without it! For example, when I ran a marathon in Prague in 2009, lying on this mat for eight minutes twice a day set my biological time to the current time of day in Prague. Because of this device, jet lag was less of a problem. We love this product and stand by it 7 years later! Visit: http://robenson.swissbionic.com or call (505) 986-1089 for more information.

STATIC VS. PULSATING TECHNOLOGY

Out of all of the technology I have tested personally and professionally in my practice and while traveling, nothing comes close to the life-changing health benefits I have experienced and witnessed with thousands of people, more than the PEMF/MRS system. Why? I have learned that many kinds of technologies are available, from magnets to lasers, but other healing devices that are considered static fields are effective for only short periods of time. The body acclimates and does not benefit further. Instead, the MRS/PEMF technology is assimilative, which relates to the fact that our cells always need pulsating frequencies every day and until the day we stop breathing. You cannot get too much of an *assimilative* technology. In other words, once your cells get fully charged, they cannot get any more of a good thing (http://robenson.swissbionic.com).

MUSE BRAIN-SENSING HEADBAND

Muse is a headband that works as a fitness tool for the brain, helping to calm and settle your mind so you can do more with it. The headband is comfortable and lightweight; with seven sensors that measure your brain activity the same way a heart monitor measures your pulse. The activity is then converted into data that you can track on your computer or smartphone. Each time you use Muse, for as little as three minutes a session, you'll improve your concentration (choosemuse.com).

HEART MATH INNER BALANCE APP AND SENSOR

The beauty of HeartMath is that it helps to create resonance and coherence in your cells and nervous system, thus creating a healthy heart-brain connection and a more positive spirit. This is an innovative approach to improving your reaction to stress as well as giving you an insight into your shifting moods and helping you to create a more positive outlook. It keeps track of your progress by journaling your accomplishments and can share the results with others, if you wish. It plugs into your iPhone, iPad or iPod and gives you on-screen prompts that can guide you to a state of inner peace. To find out about the Inner Balance program I recommend: http://click.linksynergy.com/fs-bin/click?id=Wl4ORSD8qeM&offerid=181219.10000044&type=3&subid=0.

STRUCTURED WATER DEVICES

Structured or energized water creates increased energy and vitality. It also penetrates every cell and enhances hydration, which in turn improves every cellular process in your body. A portable device by Patrick Durkin that is handy for travel is available from this website: (https://bhe88838.isrefer.com/go/specialoffer/a172/)

NES - MiHEALTH DEVICE

NES Health has not only discovered and mapped the human body field, it has also managed to integrate this groundbreaking knowledge with the principles of energy information. MiHealth, a pocket-size device, uses bio-electro stimulation and magnetic fields to deliver the information your body needs to return to a natural state, which is where all healing begins. This cutting-edge device is capable of transmitting information to the body at frequencies that match specific parts of the body, resulting in quicker and more effective treatments (http://www.neshealth.com/total-wellnes-system/nes-mihealth/).

BIOMODULATOR BY JERRY TENNANT, M.D.

With the Tennant Biomodulator, you can assess the voltage (pH) and then switch to a treatment mode to insert electrons to raise the voltage (pH), thus helping to eliminate pain. In addition to the Biomodulator, to resolve health issues, you must raise the voltage (pH) by whatever means that allows you to insert electrons into the system, including alkaline water, ozone therapy, raw fruits and vegetables, sunshine, moving water, exercise, etc.

Mini CPAP (for sleep apnea)

I was thrilled to find out about this easy-to-travel-with CPAP machine for people with sleep apnea. While you may go on vacation, sleep apnea never does, so it stands to reason that sleep apnea sufferers should never leave home without their CPAP. The small and lightweight Transcend CPAP is an alternative to lugging around a full-size CPAP unit. The Transcend Travel CPAP allows travelers to easily bring the therapy they need to maintain the benefits of healthy sleep. Find them here at www.minicpap.com. You do need to get a prescription from your doctor for the CPAP machine.

Homing Pin

Did you know airlines mishandle over 20 million bags a year and can take up to a week or more to match the bag to its owner? Every 3.5 seconds, someone in America loses a cell phone. It's so easy to lose a laptop, camera and passport. Most found items are not returned because the owner cannot easily be located. Integrated into 2,200 airports, HomingPIN™ is the world's first truly global lost property AND RECOVERY system. Protects bags, keys, cell phones, cameras and more from loss. "The world's first global lost property recovery system."

This is simply a brilliant and easy-to-use system, to travel confidently with your important belongings. The Homing Pin is a device that tracks and allows the user to recover lost goods. Each sticker has a code on it that will track lost luggage, your phone, computer and other valuables back to you. There are a great number of lost goods such as luggage, cellphones, laptops, etc. that are never recovered during travel. The items that are retrievable can take days to recover. With Homing Pin, you are aware of the location of your personal belongings at all times, so loss recovery is virtually instantaneous. For more information on Homing Pin, visit http://www.homingpin.com/healthytraveler and enter coupon code HT2015 to receive a 20% discount.

Flight Shield

Flight Shield is a nonwoven micro-porous film that creates a safe barrier between you and the airplane seat. It is a fact that 2.3 million people fly every day and the average airplane is cleaned only every 30 days. This increases the risk of contracting multiple pathogens from something as simple and seemingly benign as a seat on an airplane. The common types of bacteria found on airplanes include cold and flu, MRSA, E. Coli, Listeria and more.

LifeStraw

The LifeStraw device enables users to safely drink water from contaminated sources. Also, there's a good cause behind this product. For every LifeStraw product purchased, a school child in a developing country is provided with safe drinking water for an entire school year. You can find LifeStraw at: www.buylifestraw.com. I love this product!

LollyZip

This is a great kit I use for my toiletries and, no, it does not leak. Excellent quality and I love the people who came up with this idea. Packing your favorite personal care is a zip with LollyZip, a sophisticated travel kit. With the original TSA-compliant travel kit, with LollyZip easy-to-fill bottles and jars, you will ZIP through packing and ZIP through airport security! Lollyzip.com

Aqua Vault: "Enjoy the sun without getting burned"

Aqua Vault is a personal safe designed to enhance your level of personal safety and comfort while enjoying the great outdoors. The stylish lock box easily and quickly attaches to furniture, strollers, etc., without costly permanent additions. You can find them at www.theaquavault.com.

Goodwipes: "The quick way to get clean"

After enduring a long, hot weekend in the Florida sun at a music festival, these guys figured they needed a quick way to get clean. The result: Goodwipes. These handy little items are a large, biodegradable, hypoallergenic body wipe you can take with you on the go. You can buy them at www.goodwipes.com.

GO Sleep USA (neck support)

Finally, a pillow, neck support system that works for passengers in planes, trains, buses and cars. I met the inventors of this system at the annual Travel Goods Show. This is the best sleep system I have seen for the Healthy Conscious Traveler. GO Sleep has released a truly effective, upright sleep system designed to allow today's busy traveler a restful sleep *"on the GO."* It includes several features such as a pillow carrying case that can be used for neck or back support. The premium sleep mask sits away from the face and allows eye movement. An adjustable elastic cord with toggles secures to the seat or adjustable headrest, comfortably supporting the head in place. To learn more, go to www.gosleepusa.net.

RESTAHEAD NECK REST: FOR TRAVEL AND RELAXATION

Restahead neck rest adapts to your neck, when you lean back against a seat or lie down. It supports your neck in an ergonomically correct position and prevents your head from rolling forward or sideways. Your muscles can relax, which gives you supreme comfort and maximum rest and helps prevent a sore neck. Find them here at www.shop.restahead.com.

YON SMART BLANKET

This smart device is perfect for the traveler. It's a wearable blanket that slips on so it stays in place and gives you mobility while you snuggle up. You can sleep during your flight with privacy, and when you arrive, within seconds you can pack the blanket away in its own carrier pouch. Get it here at www.yonsmartblanket.com.

LUMOSITY

Lumosity's scientists have created and studied the Brain Performance Test (BPT), a brief, repeatable assessment battery developed to measure performance on cognitive and neuropsychological tasks. The tasks included in the BPT were selected to measure cognitive abilities, including speed of processing, memory, attention, mental flexibility, and problem solving, but are distinct from the Lumosity training exercises. Therefore, the BPT allows us to study training-related changes in scores on the specific tasks. An analysis that included nearly 1,000 subscribers who took the BPT before and after 10 weeks of Lumosity training was presented at the 2012 Society for Neuroscience meeting. This analysis found that users who completed more Lumosity training showed larger improvements in scores on the BPT (lumosity.com/hcp/research).

PEAK

Peak delivers brain training that can improve your cognitive skills. It offers fun yet challenging games, goals and workouts. Because it is expressly designed for mobile devices, it does not involve spending long periods of time in front of a desktop computer. You can train with Peak whenever and wherever it best suits you (peak.net/index.html#section-b).

MEDITATION TAPES AND YOGA DVDS

My recommendation is to travel with the music you enjoy most to help you relax and sleep. If you love yoga, have an app or two that you can use and do yoga on the road. Here are a few that I suggest: *Music: Deep Sleep* CD by Kelly Howell; *Yoga: Yoga New Beginnings* DVD with Pasha Hogan; *One Prayer* CD by Pritpal Singh Khalsa.

Section 4: Electro-sanitizing Protocols

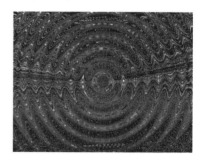

Providing protection from the assault of man-made frequencies

EARTHING SHEETS AND DEVICES

Earthing products simply conduct the actual frequencies of the earth to your body without any stimulation and serve as extension cords from the earth to you. The signal they carry includes all of the subtleties inherent in nature that our bodies have attuned to throughout history. Earthing is totally natural, as metallic materials conduct the flow of electrons. Earthing products utilize carbon or silver as the conductive agent. Silver is highly conductive and very strong, allowing it to hold up well with frequent use and washings. It is also inherently anti-microbial. Earthing products include grounding mats for computers, cars and body bands that are ideal for use while at work or while traveling, whether by car, plane, bus or train. (http://www.earthing.com/?Click=45538) Also check: http://www.bioelectricshield.com/DrBenson for a discount for the Healthy Conscious Traveler.

GENERAL EMF PROTECTION TECHNOLOGY AND PRODUCTS

Some of the websites below provide the most comprehensive overview of extraordinary technology and products that are efficient in protecting you, your family and your home from the health hazards of electro-smog. Cell phone protection, cordless phone neutralizers and other items are highly effective for minimizing radiation exposure. These can also be applied to your computer, handheld devices, hair dryers and shavers, to name a few. You can buy detergents and other household items that provide radiation shielding for all fabrics. In addition, you can find curtains and paint that shield your residence from a neighbor's Wi-Fi router running 24/7. Also, make sure to include the Protectoplex as part of your EMF personal shielding. The Protectoplex Environmental Protection holographic card serves as a baseline of strength, taking you safely through environments you can't control. Its protective field helps guard you against electromagnetic fields (EMFs), geopathic stress zones, and environmental stressors. You will find these and many other incredibly efficient products on these websites:

- www.bioelectricshield.com/DrBenson
- www.safespaceprotection.com/safespace-emf-solutions. aspx
- www.blockemf.com
- www.emfsafetystore.com

EMF PROTECTIVE CELL PHONE AND COMPUTER NEUTRALIZING STICKERS

You can view the products we sell at our healing center by visiting santafesoul.com. Although we have tried various cell phone adhesives over the years, we are now using and promoting the Aulterra brand. The efficacy of these stickers is highly controversial; however, we get mostly positive feedback. Here is where you can find the Aulterra brand stickers: https://www.aulterra.com/.

EMF PROTECTIVE NECKLACES, BRACELETS, AND OTHER BODY ITEMS

Our number-one choice for a protective necklace can be found at bioelectricshield.com/DrBenson. You can still listen to Virginia Brown's profound interview regarding the bioelectric shield at: healthytravelerssummit.com. To view this device, go to bioelectricshield.com/DrBenson.

THE QUANTUM COMPANION

This device creates harmonic fields around the body to help relieve the disruption of our biological system from the inevitable electrosmog. It attaches to your clothes or belt and looks identical to a pager. I always have this attached to my clothing when I travel, and I put it bedside while I sleep at night. This company also makes automobile products to support you when traveling by car (quantumproducts.com).

WEIN COMPANY AIR SUPPLY MINI-MATE WEARABLE AIR PURIFIERS

This is top of the line in personal air purification devices. It's light, only one and a half ounces, and purifies your breathing space. This company also provides room and auto ionizers (weinproducts.com/frontpage.htm).

FOR MOTHERS-TO-BE

The past 25 years of research has identified several potential health hazards during pregnancy from radiation, including birth defects and genetic disruptions, miscarriages, autism, childhood leukemia and cancer. Because scientists have shown that cell growth and DNA replication are disrupted by radiation, pregnancy and early childhood represent the highest risk for exposure. Please check these three websites to find clothing that can protect you and your baby:

- http://www.bellyarmor.com/
- mummywraps.com
- http://lessemf.com/index.html

WOMEN'S AND MEN'S PROTECTIVE UNDERWEAR

Swiss clothing manufacturer Isa Bodywear has launched a special line of men's underwear that claims to protect "men's sperm from harmful cell phone radiation." The briefs are made with threads of silver, which the company claims block cell phone rays and reception. The inventor, Andreas Sallmann, says that when you put a cell phone inside your briefs and then dial your number from another phone, you probably won't even get a signal (isabodywear.ch).

STETZERIZER

This highly effective electrical outlet filter reduces the dirty electricity that can leak into your home, especially in the restorative places like your bedroom. The stetzerizer also delivers a meter that can detect how much dirty electricity emanates from your electrical outlets. I personally recommend these filters for home and office use. For a 2,000 square-foot house, plan to spend between $600 and $1,000 to neutralize your living space. This is one of several different electro-sanitizing efforts we have put into place at our healing center, Santa Fe Soul (www.santafesoul.com), to ensure that our patients are getting the best possible health care, and also to protect our support staff and practitioners. This helps us all with our moods, memory and our overall energy throughout the day. Prior to these electro-sanitizing changes, many of our electro-sensitive patients and practitioners felt unwell when in our center. Indoor pollution and its health ramifications are an ever-increasing problem (stetzerizer-us.com).

EMF METER

This meter is one of the best investments you can make in your travel, home and health care needs. When you use this meter, it detects harmful, artificial frequencies. Please know, there are lots of choices on the web. *Not to be repetitive, but this will be one of the best investments you make, not only in your personal and travel life, but for your whole family.* Check every outlet, wall space, and appliance you have for high EMF and microwave smog. Notice the high EMF output from dimmer switches and all outlets. Ouch! Just hear the hissing noise that is all around you that without this device you never hear, smell or taste. HD TVs are off the chart, as are most light fixtures, hair dryers, electric shavers and, yes, even vacuum cleaners. One patient of mine took home our office EMF meter. After sweeping her home, she was utterly blown away to discover that behind the wall where her son slept was a huge electrical panel for the house. Finally, she discovered why her 14-year-old son was suffering from severe insomnia and frequent colds. She moved his bed to a healthy EMF zone in the same room and his health and sleep patterns improved immediately. You can purchase an EMF meter at www.jointheselfcarerevolution.com/deep-healing-frequencies/ or lessemf.com/rf.html#481 or call our office at 505-986-1089 to order the one we use.

Buy a low-radiation phone

When you pick up your phone and make a call, that call is transmitted and received via the phenomena of electromagnetic waves. Newer and more advanced phones, such as the more popular smartphone models, are being developed with increasing degrees of cell phone radiation emissions. Consult the buyer's guide for a low-emission phone and consider replacing yours with one that they recommend in the *EWG Buyer's Guide*: ewg.org/cellphoneradiation/ Get-a-Safer-Phone.

Choose texting over talking

Research has confirmed that during transmission time (call time), a considerable amount of radiation travels inward toward the ear and head of the cell phone user. Several recent studies show a correlation between cell phone radiation emission and conditions involving the brain or within the region of the head. The Environmental Working Group (EWG) reports this:

Brain Cancer: Two analyses of 25 original publications identified a 50% to 90% increase in risk for two types of brain tumors: glioma and acoustic neuroma.(4)

Salivary Gland Tumors: An Israeli study found an increased risk of 50% to 60% for salivary gland tumors among people with the highest cell phone use.(5)

Behavioral Problems: A study of 13,159 Danish children showed an 80% elevated risk for emotional and hyperactivity problems among young children who used cell phones and whose mothers also used cell phones during pregnancy.(6)

Migraines and Vertigo: A study of 420,095 Danish adults showed that long-term cell phone users were 10% to 20% more likely to be hospitalized for migraines and vertigo than people who took up cell phones more recently.(7)

Of the total radiation emitted towards the head, 97% to 99% is absorbed into the hemisphere of the brain on the side where the cell phone is used. Which area generally receives the highest radiation exposure? The temporal lobe. This area is involved in hearing, auditory processing, formation of long-term memory, speech and vision.(8)

If a phone is worn near the waist, as is often the case when a headset is used, the outgoing radiation is absorbed by the soft tissue located there and could also cause health issues.(9)

USE A HEADSET OR SPEAKER

Keep the phone away from the body. The latest research is still in debate on whether wireless or corded headsets are better for your health. A wireless tube headset device was developed recently that uses a patented sound delivery process allowing sound to travel through an air-filled wireless tube. Here is a reputable manufacturer of safe headsets: smart-safe.com/.

CHILDREN AND CELL PHONES: LIMIT YOUR CHILD'S PHONE USE!

Children are more sensitive to cell phone radiation emissions than adults because their bone tissue is less dense. Additionally, the brain of a child is still developing, and its nervous tissue can absorb a greater amount of radiation than an adult. Research by French Telecom scientists showed that under standard conditions of use, twice as much cell phone radiation would penetrate a child's thinner, softer skull than an adult's, making them more susceptible to brain tumors. These results confirm earlier findings, from 1996 and 2002, that a child's head absorbs more radio frequency radiation than an adult.(10) The research surrounding children and health risks associated with cell phone use is staggering. Yes, you may agree strongly that cell phones for children are a great "safety" tool. This is true if used only in emergency situations and by also following safety guideline such as texting instead of calling, and keeping the phone away from your ear by using the speakerphone function.

Health agencies in France, Germany, Israel, Switzerland and the United Kingdom have recommended reducing children's exposure to cell phone radiation. Researchers in Sweden found the highest risk of brain tumors among people who started using cell phones during adolescence.(11)

In a nutshell: keep your kids away from cell phones. If you are pregnant, consider eliminating cell phone use as much as possible, and also keep laptops off your lap.

PREVENTATIVE ACTION STEPS WITH PHONES

- Text instead of talking as often as possible.
- Use an approved speakerphone or a headset, and keep your phone away from your body.
- Use functional wear and accessories.
- Only use your phone if you have a strong signal.
- Limit your child's cell phone use. Dr. Mehmet Oz recommends limiting use until your child is 15 years old.
- Never charge your phone when it is near your head. It is best to charge in another room while your phone is turned off.
- ***Join the Allstate Insurance - xthetext campaign on Facebook and encourage your friends not to text and drive.

ELECTRO-SANITIZE YOUR HOME, WORKPLACE AND HOTEL WITH INTELLIGENT TECHNOLOGY

- Hire an EMF Clean Sweep agent (www.EMFCleanSweep.com).
- Invest in stetzerizer plugs that go into outlets and neutralize EMFs.
- Invest in a Smart Meter EMF encasing.
- Invest in an EMF meter detector (listed above).
- Invest in the IMRS mat(http://robenson.swissbionic.com).
- Relocate your Wi-Fi router as far away from the bedroom area as possible.
- Unplug all electrical equipment in your hotel before bedtime.

- Relocate baby monitors as far away from the crib as possible.

- If residing in row housing or an apartment building, educate your neighbors on the effects of EMF, and ask them to turn off their Wi-Fi at night.

- Utilize earthing products to protect your home and travel environment from neighboring rooms or the home's electro-smog.

- Unplug the microwave and other electrical items in the kitchen when not in use.

- Omit the use of microwaves and wireless phones, major culprits in high radiation even when not in use yet plugged in. I discovered this when I used my EMF gauss meter for the first time in my home. I was shocked to see how much radiation was emitting from our microwave that was plugged in, but not in use. Yes, that was the last time we ever used a microwave in our house.

- Space Safe II is perfect for bedrooms or office spaces, as it is effective in clearing, re-energizing and balancing energies for EMF protection in a nine-foot radius. (safespaceprotection .com/products/emf-protection-home-office-safespace)

For a very informative site regarding the unseen environmental causes for your affected ailments, visit: bewellbuzz.com/ wellness-buzz/7-hidden-dangers-home.

WHEN TRAVELING BY AUTOMOBILE

- Purchase a grounding rod for your car. This minimizes the static and radiation while driving. You can order it from the Earthing company.

- Purchase a Space Safe II for your car, which is effective in clearing, re-energizing and balancing energies for EMF protection in a nine-foot radius.

- Purchase an air-ionizer for your car, as it is safer than the highly toxic "air fresheners."

- When you buy a new car, allow it to air out/off-gas for days before you drive it. When getting your car cleaned and detailed, ask for environmentally friendly products. Maintain air circulation in your car at all times, even in the winter. You can crack a window a bit. EMFs are intensified by the car's radio bands, the use of cellphones and when your GPS is engaged.

- Cell phones draw more power and emit more radiation in enclosed metal spaces. (experiencelife.com)
- Use a Bluetooth/tube headset while driving.
- Consume one 8-ounce glass of water per driving hour. Increased hydration equals healthier cells and increased cellular voltage equals decreased EMF effects.

Section 5: Travel Health Tips and Recommended Therapies

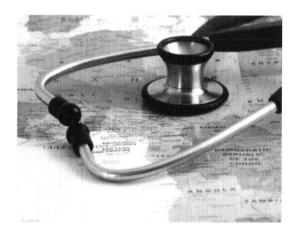

A healthy immune system is key to the success of your travel experience. The following are treatments, along with other health travel tips, that help support your immune system.

To listen to 35 acclaimed health and travel experts talk about how to stay healthy with travel, visit www.healthytravelerssummit.com.

If you would like to engage with my health center and a group of self-care coaches to help you with any health concerns, please contact Santa Fe Soul Center for Optimal Health at santafesoul.

com and join our global, free online program to stay tuned with top health experts and wellness news (jointheselfcarerevolution.com). Or join us for a life-promoting five-day retreat for revitalization or to overcome a chronic health challenge (freshstartsantafe.com).

Chinese Acupuncture: Chinese medicine is one of the oldest forms of medicine, and it dates back millennia. Western medicine, in contrast, has only been around for the past 200 years. Acupuncture treatments aim to balance energy meridians, allowing the body to heal itself. Relatively painless, it is administered by inserting fine needles at key points on the body relating to various organs. I treat just about any known health challenge with acupuncture, and since I live in Santa Fe, which is a travel destination, I treat travelers from all over the world. For relief from jet lag, altitude sickness, sciatica, neck pain and more, acupuncture and Chinese herbs are always an excellent choice.

Chiropractic Adjustments: Great to do before and after long travel, especially if you have spinal and nutritional imbalances, including sciatica and neck pain. "Prolonged sitting can wreak havoc on your body," says Dr. Scott Bautch, an American Chiropractic Association (ACA) media spokesperson. "Even if you travel in the most comfortable car or opt to fly first class, certain pressures and forces from awkward positions can result in restricted blood flow."

Myers Cocktail: This intravenous treatment (vitamin C, magnesium, calcium, vitamins B12, B6 and more) is best used for an immune boost, taken before or after travel to treat adrenal fatigue and low energy, depression, fibromyalgia and vitamin deficiencies. It's also great for sports performance enhancement and an overall lift in your spirits.

Ultraviolet Blood Irradiation (UVB): For more than 100 years, this light therapy treatment has been used for a variety of medical conditions. The procedure involves removing about 60 cc of blood (the amount in a typical glass of water) and passing the blood through a quartz cuvette, where it is exposed to ultraviolet light and returned to the blood stream. The ultraviolet light used is the same wave length produced by sunlight. Check out my website for more information, robynbenson.com. This is a very popular procedure that many medical tourists seek. Listen to my interview with John Cote of Healthcare Elsewhere to learn more (http://healthcareelsewhere.com/?s=robyn+benson).

B12 Shots: Vitamin B12 (cobalamin) is an essential water-soluble vitamin used by the body to maintain healthy nerve cells, produce RNA, DNA and red blood cells and to help iron function properly. B12 also works with folate to produce the amino acid SAMe, which controls mood and supports immune function. B12 injections have many benefits and are often prescribed for deficiencies that cause fatigue, shortness of breath, diarrhea, numbness and neurological damage.

Intravenous Vitamin C : Vitamin C is needed for healthy gums, to help protect against infection and to aid with clearing up infections. Vitamin C is thought to enhance the immune system, lower high blood pressure and prevent arteriosclerosis (http://robynbenson.com/santa-fe-soul/). IV C is also common in many chronic illness protocols as well.

Massage: Massage offers more than just caring and comfort. According to the Mayo Clinic, studies demonstrate that it is an effective treatment for reducing stress, pain and muscle tension. Some studies have found massage to be helpful for anxiety, insomnia, digestive disorders and headaches—all conditions that the traveler can experience.

Platelet Rich Plasma (PRP): PRP is a prolotherapy injection procedure that uses the platelets in a patient's blood to help mend serious injuries, decrease the time for healing and ultimately decrease the overall need for surgery. It is also used as a skin rejuvenation therapy, which aids in reducing wrinkles, tightens the skin, and brings about general improvement in skin texture (robynbenson.com).

Prolozone: Prolozone is a form of non-surgical ligament reconstruction that is often a treatment for chronic pain. By repairing the connective tissue, this is all that is needed to permanently reverse chronic pain in many cases. Prolozone Therapy is an injection technique similar to prolotherapy but uses ozone. This is one of my absolute favorite therapies that I give each day to my patients. It is easy to administer, not too painful, cost effective and best of all, it works! Often just one to three injections can help repair an injured knee. To find out more, and the research behind this therapy, visit http://santafesoul.com/services/prolozone-therapy/.

Photon Genius: This instrument communicates with all the cells of the body to balance and enliven all systems and organs of the body. It's the first and only instrument in the world combining the genius of Ed Skilling with sophisticated, proprietary circuitry, generating the genius dynamics of Photon-Genetic Energy, Life-force Energy Transmission, Harmonic Frequency Tube Technology and Harmonic Infrared Energy Transmission. Patients come from near and far to use our Photon Genius, because we are the only center in New Mexico that has one. Excellent for chronic health issues.

Cold Laser: In this non-thermal, noninvasive treatment, a cold laser is used to treat chronic and acute pain and inflammation. This therapy also promotes higher serotonin levels, which helps the body heal. I often use my cold laser on open wounds, nerve issues and for any type of dental pain and trauma.

Far Infrared Sauna (FIR): FIR infrared ray energy is part of the natural light spectrum, minus the skin-damaging effects of UV rays. The many benefits of this sauna include weight loss, improved metabolism, increased energy, decreased stress, elevated immune function, better circulation, detoxification of the body, and purification of the skin.

EFT: The Emotional Freedom Technique, or EFT, is a psychological acupressure technique known as "tapping" that can optimize your emotional health and help reduce fear of flying and other negative travel-related emotions.

Mindfulness Practice: The practice of focusing your attention solely on the present moment with no judgment, mindfulness has been identified as key component of happiness that improves both physical and mental health.

Meditation: Meditation, whether sitting or walking, is one of your best choices for mental fitness. It is relaxing and it also teaches your mind to focus and allows you to be more resilient with the unexpected during travel and in daily life.

Minute Suites: Minute Suites offer travelers in airports a private retreat where they can nap, relax or work. It's a great place to unwind during a long trip, as each suite includes a daybed sofa and a sound-masking system to neutralize noise. There's even a unique audio program to help you sleep and an alarm clock to make sure you don't miss your plane! Presently, these suites can be found at these airports: Hartsfield-Jackson Atlanta International, Philadelphia International and Dallas-Fort Worth International (minutesuites.com).

Natural Spring Waters: "Find a Spring" is a community-creat-ed database and map of natural spring water sources all over the world! Minerals like lithium, magnesium, sulfur and calcium, all found in spring water, can have therapeutic effects on skin diseases and infections like psoriasis and dermatitis. Bathing in spring water can also be a preventative treatment and protection against blood diseases, nutritional disorders, and chronic digestive disorders. It has also been known to provide holistic treatment for hypertension and other heart and lung problems. Also, I am a big fan of drinking water from natural springs around the world. Check out a place close to you (findaspring.com).

Ecotourism: Traveling to natural areas that are pristine, often fragile and relatively untouched by humans is the focus of eco-tourism, which stresses socially responsible travel. The goal may be to educate the traveler, to contribute to the economic develop-ment of a local community or even to financially support ecological conservation. Ecotourism involves travel to destinations prized for their cultural heritage, as well as for their flora and fauna. Travelers will gain insight into how humans impact the natural environment and also increase their appreciation of the world's natural habi-tats. To learn more, visit these links: the world's oldest and largest ecotourism association: http://www.ecotourism.org/; a directory of the world's accredited ecotourism resorts: http://www.eco-tropical resorts.com/.

MEDICAL TRAVEL PLANNING/RESOURCES/SAFETY

Medical Tourism: There's a growing trend of people around the world traveling to other countries to receive health care, primarily because it is less expensive and has a shorter wait time but also be-cause some procedures aren't available in the countries where they live. A 2014 estimate shows that more than 1.2 million Americans took medical trips that year, and that number is only expected to grow, especially as the world's population ages.(13)

John Cote, a pilot and the creator and host of *Healthcare Elsewhere*, a medical tourism show and podcast, interviews doctors, health care experts and patients worldwide who travel to foreign countries to receive treatments that are either too expensive or not available in the U.S. It's all about educating people globally about opportunities that exist for them to travel and receive world-class health care at affordable prices. Cote has also authored the best-selling books *Healthcare Elsewhere* and *Mobilize Your Customers* and is currently writing *Onwards* with co-author Ron Phillips. To listen to my interview on John Cote's show click here: (itunes.apple.com/us/podcast/healthcare-elsewhere-medical/id865339093) Episode 105. John Cote is also one of the featured speakers in www.healthytravelerssummit.com.

Protect Your Valuables with the Homingpin System: See above! (http://www.homingpin.com/.)

STEPS FOR MEDICAL TRAVEL

1. Always obtain copies of all your lab tests and radiology reports that are necessary.

2. Have a thorough check-up with your doctor before travel.

3. Create a folder for your personal health and wellness profile.

4. If you can, scan your medical documents and save in PDF format, and/or store on your phone for easy access. You just never know what can happen, HCT, so be prepared!

ANNUAL BLOOD TESTS ARE ADVISED FOR ALL HCTS

The HCT knows the importance of having an annual blood test that includes chem screen, HDL, CBC, a full thyroid panel, hormone panel, vitamin D3 levels, C-reactive protein and homocysteine levels. Consider adding blood mercury and lead levels, too. For an accurate assessment of Heavy Metal Burden, work with a qualified physician who can offer a six-hour urine test through a reputable lab. To find out if you have celiac disease or gluten sensitivity, I recommend Cyrex labs. For a general food sensitivity test, I use US Biotek Labs for my patients (US BioTek Laboratories http://www.usbiotek.com/index.html; Doctor's Data https://www.doctorsdata.com (heavy metals, stool tests).

Vaccination and Travel: Getting vaccinated is a personal health choice, however some vaccines are mandatory to enter a country. Only you can decide what is right for you and your family. Always check the vaccine requirements of every country you plan to visit. I had to get the yellow fever vaccination when I traveled to Kenya.

I chose not to take the pills for malaria, and I am one lucky girl. To this day, I have never had malaria. Instead I have taken homeopathic tinctures infused with these possible pathogens. By taking these in homeopathic form, I am ingesting minute amounts of the pathogen in order to allow my immune system to not recognize the bug as a foreigner.

So far, this has worked well for me. Even though antimalarial drugs have some nasty side effects, getting malaria can be deadly, so make sure you work with a holistic practitioner who is well-versed in this subject and who can offer an alternative for you. To view alternatives to malaria pills and the best herbs to take while traveling, see Chapter 9.

Lodging, Dining and Shopping: Check www.yelp.com or ask your hotel concierge to find the closest health food stores and organic restaurants. Just log on and search for your dining preference, be it vegetarian, vegan, raw, bar and grill, etc. You will also be able to find natural foods markets near your lodging location. It would also be a good idea to locate spas, hotels, health practitioners and medical offices.

Natural and Organic Products at Reduced Prices for the HCT: Thrive Market is the first socially conscious online store offering the world's best-selling natural and organic products at wholesale prices. They carry more than 2,500 of the highest quality food, supplements, home and personal care and beauty products from more than 400 of the best brands on the market, all delivered straight to your door at 25% to 50% off retail prices. Thrives's mission is to make healthy living easy, affordable and accessible for every American family https://thrivemarket.com/affiliates?affiliate_id=3424.

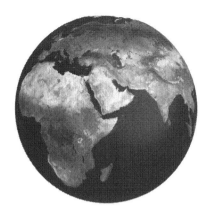

Epilogue

We've arrived at the end of our journey together as Healthy Conscious Travelers. We've explored so much territory and learned about many travel tools and tips.

You are now ready to roam the world with the knowledge of how to travel healthy and stress-free, how to eat right and keep fit and how to enjoy a happy and safe trip.

Know that by following The 8 Pathways as outlined in these pages, you're ensuring that wherever you travel and by whatever means, you'll arrive refreshed and ready for adventure! And if you eat the foods that promote vibrant health, sleep well and take the steps to protect yourself from travel pollution, your journey will be an easy one, health wise, and you'll be in top shape to enjoy your travels.

Be sure to check out the resources included in this book (Chapter 10), as you will find state-of-the-art equipment, unique tools for travel, health supplements and vitamins, recommended books, films and blogs and much more.

Also, pick up a copy of *The Healthy Conscious Traveler's Food Guide* (www.robynbenson.com) for great recipes and tips on home-made foods for travel. You'll also want a copy of *The Healthy Conscious Traveler's First Aid Kit*, filled with essential oils for health, vitamins and supplements and much more to keep you on the path to health and wellness, no matter where you go!

Now that you've learned how to become a Healthy Conscious Traveler, test your knowledge by taking the Healthy Conscious Traveler's Quiz (Appendix A). There are 200 additional questions at www.robyn benson.com.

Thanks for taking this journey with me, HTC. Much love and happy trails to you.

Dr. Robyn Benson http://robynbenson.com/

Founder of Santa Fe Soul Center for Optimal Health http://santa fesoul.com/

Founder of the Self-Care Revolution http://jointheselfcare revolution.com/

Creator of the Healthy Conscious Traveler's Global Summit http:// healthytravelerssummit.com/

Endnotes

Introduction

1. Alex Matsuo, "Trillion Dollar Zeitgeist: The World's 10 Richest Industries," TheRichest.com, 14 Jan., 2014. http://www.the richest.com/rich-list/world/trillion-dollar-zeitgeist-the-worlds-10-richest-industries/.

2. Air Transport Action Group, "Aviation: Benefits Beyond Borders," April 2014. http://aviationbenefits.org/media/26786/ATAG_AviationBenefits2014_FULL_LowRes.pdf.

3. U.S. Department of Energy, "About Radiation," 2012. http://www.epa.gov/radiation/docs/402-k-10-008.pdf.

4. Patrick Smith's Ask the Pilot, "The Truth About Cabin Air," http://www.askthepilot.com/questionanswers/cabin-air-quality/.

5. S. Humphreys et al., "The Effect of High Altitude Commercial Air Travel on Oxygen Saturation," *Anaesthesia*, May 2005. http://www.ncbi.nlm.nih.gov/pubmed/15819766.

6. Homingpin.com, http://www.homingpin.com/.

Chapter 1

1. Mark Hyman, M.D., "Is There Toxic Waste in You Body" DrHyman.com, 8 May, 2013, http://drhyman.com/blog/2010/05/19/is-there-toxic-waste-in-your-body-2/#close.

Chapter 2

1. "George Washington University report calculates the financial cost of being obese," *Washington Post*, 21 Sept. 2010, http://

www.washingtonpost.com/wp-dyn/content/article/2010/09/20/AR2010092004738.html.

2. Elisabeth Rosenthal, "Even Small Medical Advances Can Mean Big Jumps in Bills," *The New York Times*, 5 April 2014, http://www.nytimes.com/2014/04/06/health/even-small-medical-advances-can-mean-big-jumps-in-bills.html.

3. Dr. Hyman "Eat Your Medicine: Food As Pharmacology," DrHyman.com, 14 Oct. 2014, http://drhyman.com/blog/2011/10/14/eat-your-medicine-food-as-pharmacology/.

4. American Heart Association, "Fish 101," Heart.org, http://www.heart.org/HEARTORG/GettingHealthy/NutritionCenter/Fish-101_UCM_305986_Article.jsp.

5. Robynne K. Chutkan, MD, "Could Leaky Gut Be What's Troubling You?" DoctorOz.com, 20 Feb. 2013, http://www.doctoroz.com/article/could-leaky-gut-be-troubling-you.

Chapter 3

1. Fr. Booth., et al. "Waging war on modern chronic diseases: primary prevention through exercise biology." *Journal of Applied Physiology*. Vol. 88, Issue 2, pp. 774-787, February 2010, http://jap.physiology.org/content/88/2/774.

2. J. Thompson Coon, et al., "Does Participating in Physical Activity in Outdoor Natural Environments Have a Greater Effect on Physical and Mental Wellbeing than Physical Activity Indoors? A Systematic Review," *Environmental Science & Technology*, 3 Feb. 2011, http://pubs.acs.org/doi/abs/10.1021/es102947t.

3. Mayo Clinic Staff, "Pilates for beginners, Explore the Core, MayoClinic.org, 5 Feb. 2014, http://www.mayoclinic.org/healthy-lifestyle/fitness/in-depth/pilates-for-beginners/art-20047673.

4. Join the Self-Cafe Revolution, JoinTheSelfCareRevolution.com, http://www.jointheselfcarerevolution.com/the-self-care-revolution-package/.

Chapter 4

1. Masaru Emoto, Masaru-Emoto.net, http://www.masaru-emoto .net/english/emoto.html.

2. S. Humphreys et al., "The effect of high altitude commercial air travel on oxygen saturation," *Aeneasthesia*, May 2005, http://www. ncbi.nlm.nih.gov/pubmed/15819766.

3. Jerry Tennant, *Healing is Voltage*, CreateSpace Independent Publishing Platform, 2010.

4. Kona Sea Salt, KonaSeaSalt.com. http://www.konaseasalt.com/ index.php/about-kona-sea-salt/hawaii-sea-salt-and-your%20 health/206.

5. David Rosenfield, David, "How a personal experience led to the creation of a worldwide vitamin company," *Westside People*, February 2015, http://www.westsidepeoplemag.com/2015/02/ oxylent-lisa-lent-vitamins/.

6. Joseph Mercola, "Is Your Water Safe?" http://www.mercola.com/ downloads/bonus/chlorine/default.htm.

7. Jenn Bilbrey, "BPA-Free Plastic Containers May Be Just as Hazardous," *Scientific American*, 11 August 2014, http://www.scien tificamerican.com/article/bpa-free-plastic-containers-may-be- just-as-hazardous/.

8. Ibid.

9. Adam Abraham, "Shedding More Light on Structured Water, *Phaelosopher*, 19 Feb. 2010, http://phaelosopher.com/2010/02/19/ shedding-more-light-on-structured-water/.

10. Natural Actions Technologies (2014). Water Products. http:// naturalactiontechnologies.com/products/.

11. Kona Sea Salt, konaseasalt.com, www.konaseasalt.com/ index.php/about-kona-sea-salt/hawaii-sea-salt-and-your health/206.

12. Charity Water, ChariityWater.com, https://donate.charitywater.
org/donate/nepal.

Chapter 5

1. Dr. Dave's Best, http://www.drdavesbest.com/dr-daves-product-
list.html.

2. Jessica Firger, "Chronic Sleep Deprivation Linked to
Child Obesity", CBS News, 19 May, 2014, http://www.cbs
news.com/news/chronic-sleep-deprivation-linked-to-
childhood-obesity/.

3. Drowsy Driving, drowsydriving.org, http://drowsydriving.org/
about/facts-and-stats/.

4. Statistic Brain, StatisticBrain.com, http://www.statisticbrain.
com/sleeping-disorder-statistics/.

5. Pat Doyle, "Flight attendant fatigue poses safety risks."
Star Tribune, May 28, 2013. http://www.startribune.com/lo-
cal/208961821.html.

6. Easy Wake," Importance of deep sleep and REM sleep," http://
www.easywake.me/articles/importance.

7. Malka N. Halgamuge, " Pineal Melatonin Level Disruption In
Humans Due To Electromagnetic Fields And Icnirp Limits," *Oxford
Journal*, 4 Sept. 2012, http://rpd.oxfordjournals.org/content/ear-
ly/2012/10/09/rpd.ncs255.abstract.

8. Louise Ann Gittleman, "Lose Weight While You're Asleep,"
AnnLouise.com, 10 August, 2012. http://www.annlouise.com/
articles/494.

9. Earthing Institute, EarthingInstitute.net, http://www.earthingin-
stitute.net/?page_id=131.

10. Christine Horner, "25 Breast Health Tips," DrChristineHorner.
com, http://www.drchristinehorner.com/25tips.html.

Chapter 6

1. Paul Rosch, "America's Leading Adult Health Problem," *USA Magazine*, May 1991, http://www.stress.org/americas-1-health-problem/.

2. Amen Clinics, AmenClinics.com, http://store.amenclinics.com/high-performance-brains.

3. Clint Ober, et al., *Earthing: The Most Important Health Discovery Ever?*, Laguna Beach, California: Basic Health Publications, 2010, 82.

4. Pamela Weintraub, "Wake Up Call," ExperienceLife.com, Dec. 2011. https://experiencelife.com/article/wake-up-call/.

5. Ibid.

6. Cellular Phone Task Force, "Statements by Physicians, Scientists and Health Policy Experts, CellularPhoneTaskForce.com, http://www.cellphonetaskforce.org/?page_id=766.

7. Geil Browning, "10 Ways to Rejuvenate Your Brain While You Work," Inc.com, 10 Sept. 2012, http://www.inc.com/geil-browning/personal-productivity-refresh-your-brain-while-you-work.html.

8. Sheila G. Klauer, Ph.D., et. al., "Distracted Driving and Risk of Road Crashes among Novice and Experienced Drivers," *New England Journal of Medicine*, 2 Jan., 2014, http://www.nejm.org/doi/full/10.1056/NEJMsa1204142.

9. National Center for Contemplatory and Integrative Health, "Omega-3 Supplements: An Introduction," nccih.nih.gov, https://nccih.nih.gov/health/omega3/introduction.htm.

10. Daniel Amen MD, "12 Prescriptions for Creating a Brain Healthy Life," AmenClincis.com, http://www.amenclinics.com/cybcyb/12-prescriptions-for-creating-a-brain-healthy-life/.

Chapter 7

1. World Health Organization workshop on electromagnetic

hypersensitivity, October 25 -27, 2004 Prague, Czech Republic, Who.int, http://www.who.int/peh-emf/en/.

2. Susan Parsons, "Living with Electro-hypersensitivity," WeepIniti ative.org. http://www.weepinitiative.org/livingwithEHS.html.

3. Op Cit., WHO workshop on electromagnetic hypersensitivity.

4. Elaine N. Aron, PhD, *The Highly Sensitive Person: How to Thrive When The World Overwhelms You*, New York: Broadway Books, 1997, XX.

Chapter 8

1. Martin Zucker, "Earthing: The Most Important Health Discovery Ever?" TownsendLetter.com, May 2010. http://www.townsendletter. com/May2010/earthing0510.html.

2. Talia Fuhrman, "BPA: How to Avoid This Ubiquitous Chemical Menace," Diseaseproof.com, 2 Oct. 2012, http://www.diseaseproof. com/archives/cancer-bpa-how-to-avoid-this-ubiquitous-chemical- menace.html.

Chapter 9

1. The Tapping Solution, TheTappingSolution.com, http://www. thetappingsolution.com/.

2. Stop Jet Lag, StopJetLag.com, http://www.stopjetlag.com.

3. *AARP The Magazine*, April 2004, pg. 24.

4. Mark Stengler, M.D., "Dr. Stengler's Cold and Flu Protection Plan," 1 BottomLineHealth.com, 1 Oct. 2012, http://bottomlinehealth. com/dr-stenglers-cold-and-flu-protection-plan/.

5. Joseph Mercola, MD, "Astaxanthin—Nature's Most Powerful Antioxidant," Mercola.com, 10 Feb. 2013, http://shop.mercola.com/ catalog/astaxanthin,7,0,0.htm.

6. Nava Atlas, "7 Top Health Benefits of Maca," VegKitchen.com, http://www.vegkitchen.com/?s=7+top+health+benefits/.

7. Joseph Mercola, MD, "5 Grams Daily of Spirulina REVERSED Severe Radiation Poisoning in Chernobyl Children," Mercola. com, 9 Nov. 2011, http://articles.mercola.com/sites/articles/archive/2011/11/09/spirulina-reversed- radiation-damage-in-chernobyl-children-in-just-20-days.aspx.

Chapter 10

1. Mehmet Oz MD, "Ask Your Doctor About: Pulsed Electromagnetic Field Therapy," Doctoroz.com, http://www.doctoroz.com/article/ask-your-doctor-about-pulsed-electromagnetic-field-therapy.

2. Joseph L. Hardy et al., "Enhancing visual attention and working memory with a Web- based cognitive training program, *Mensa Journal*, Vol. 42 (2), Summer 2011, http://static.sl.lumosity.com/pdf/hardy_drescher_sarkar_kellet_scanlon_2011.pdf.

3. Israel New Agency, http://www.israelnewsagency.com/antistaticemfesdfireresistantmaterialsgarments5591025.html.

4. VG Khurana et al., "Cell phones and brain tumors: a review including the long-term epidemiologic data." *Surgical Neurology*, 27 March, 2009, http://www.ncbi.nlm.nih.gov/pubmed/19328536.

5. S. Sadetzki et al., "Cellular phone use and risk of benign and malignant parotid gland tumors—a nationwide case-control study," *American Journal of Epidemiology*, 6 Dec., 2011, http://www.ncbi.nlm.nih.gov/pubmed/18063591.

6. H.A. Divan et al., "Prenatal and postnatal exposure to cell phone use and behavioral problems in children," *Epidemiology*, July 2008, http://www.ncbi.nlm.nih.gov/pubmed/18467962.

7. Joachim Shüz et al., "Risks for Central Nervous System Diseases among Mobile Phone Subscribers: A Danish Retrospective Cohort Study," ncbi.nlm.nih.gov, 5 Feb. 2009, http://www.ncbi.nlm.nih.gov/pmc/articles/PMC2632742/.

8. S. Sadetzki et al., "Cellular phone use and risk of benign and malignant parotid gland tumors—a nationwide case-control study," *American Journal of Epidemiology*, 15 Feb., 2008, http://www.ncbi. nlm.nih.gov/pubmed/18063591.

9. Body Ecology, "Five Cell Phone Radiation Protection Tips," Body Ecology.com, http://bodyecology.com/articles/5-cell-phone-radiation-tips.

10. Environmental Working Group, "Cell Phone Radiation Depends on Wireless Carrier, EWG.org, 12 Nov., 2013, http://www.ewg.org/ research/cell-phone-radiation-depends-wireless-carrier.

11. Denis Aydin et al., "Mobile Phone Use and Brain Tumors in Children and Adolescents: A Multicenter Case–Control Study," *Journal of the National Cancer Institute*, 7 June, 2011 http://jnci. oxfordjournals.org/content/early/2011/07/27/jnci.djr244.abstract.

12. American Chiropractic Association, "Travel Aches and Strains Can Be a Pain in Your Back," ACAToday.com, https://www.acatoday. org/content_css.cfm?CID=92.

13. Patients Beyond Borders, PatientsBeyondBorders.com, http:// www.patientsbeyondborders.com/medical-tourism-statistics-facts.

Bibliography

Books

Aron, Elaine N. *The Highly Sensitive Person: How to Thrive When the World Overwhelms You.* New York: Carol Publishing Group, 1996.

Batmanghelidj, Fereydoon. *Your Body's Many Cries for Water.* Virginia: Global Health Solutions, Inc., 1997.

Burchard, Brendon. *The Charge: Activating the 10 Human Drives That Make You Feel Alive.* New York: Free Press, 2012.

Campbell, Colin. *China Study.* Texas: BenBella Books, 2005.

Christianson, Alan. *The Adrenal Reset Diet.* New York: Harmony Books, 2014.

Diamandis, Peter and Kotler, Steven. *Abundance: The Future is Better than You Think.* New York: Free Press, 2014.

Fairechild, Diana. *Jet Smart.* New York: Flyana.Com, 1999.

Gelb, Michael. *Brain Power: Improve Your Mind As You Age.* California: New World Library, 2012.

Gittleman, Ann Louise. *Zapped.* New York: HarperCollins Publication, 2010.

Gottfried, Sara. *The Hormone Cure.* New York: Scribner, 2013.

Gottfried, Sara. *The Hormone Reset Diet.* New York: HarperCollins Publication, 2015.

Hari, Vani. *The Food Babe Way.* New York: Little, Brown and Company, 2015.

Laporte, Paula B., et al. *Prescriptions for a Healthy House: A Practical Guide for Architects, Builders and Homeowners.* Canada: New Society Publishers, 2008.

McTaggart , Lynne. *The Field: The Quest for the Secret Force of the Universe.* New York: Free Press, 2012.

Milham, Samuel. *Dirty Electricity.* USA: iUniverse, 2010.

Ober, Clint, et al. *Earthing.* USA: Better Health Publication, 2010.

O'Connor, Bonnie Blair. *Healing Traditions, Alternative Medicine and the Health Professions.* Pennsylvania: University of Pennsylvania Press, 1995.

Singer, Katie. *An Electronic Silent Spring.* Massachusetts: Portal Books, 2014.

Tennant, Jerry. *Healing Is Voltage.* CreateSpace Independent Publishing Platform, 2010.

Werner, Eric. *The Geography of Bliss: One Grump's Search for the Happiest Places in the World.* New York: Hachette Book Group USA, 2008.

Films

Addicted to Plastic. Dir. Ian Connacher. Cryptic Moth Productions, 2008. Documentary.

Burzynski. Dir. Eric Merola. 2010. Documentary.

Fat, Sick and Nearly Dead. Dir. Joe Cross, Kurt Engfehr. Bev Pictures, 2011. Documentary.

Fed Up. Dir. Stephanie Soechtig. E1 Films Canada, 2014. Documentary.

Food Inc. Dir. Robert Kenner. Magnolia Pictures, 2009. Documentary.

Forks Over Knives. Dir. Lee Fulkerson. Monica Beach Media, 2011. Documentary.

Full Signal. Dir. Talal Jabari. Journeyman Pictures, 2010. Documentary.

Genetic Roulette: The Gamble of Our Lives. Dir. Jeffrey Smith. The Clearance Lab, 2012. Documentary.

Hungry for Change. Dir. James Colquhoun, Laurentine Bosch, Carlo Ledesma. Permacology Productions, 2012. Documentary.

Moldy. Dave Asprey. Bulletproof Media, 2015.

Origins. Dir. Pedram Shojai. Vital Origins Productions, 2014 Documentary

Thrive, What in the World Will It Take? Dir. Steve Gagnė, Kimberly Carter, Foster Gamble. Clear Compass Media, 2011. Documentary.

Unleaded. Dr. Roy Heilbron, Dr. Angelique Hart, Dir., Shereen Noon. 2012.

Vitality. Dir. Pedram Shojai. Vital Origins Productions, 2012. Documentary.

Glossary

acai berries
a small dark purple fleshy berrylike fruit of a tall slender palm (*Euterpe oleracea*) of tropical Central and South America that is often used in beverages

acetylcarnitine
a substance which can act as a carrier for acetyl groups across the inner mitochondrial membrane in mammalian liver

acidophilus
a popular term for yogurt bacteria, which help restore normal GI-tract flora, after its alteration by antibiotics; acidophilus also may be useful in managing mucocutaneous candidiasis

acoustic neuroma
a benign tumor involving cells of the myelin sheath that surrounds the vestibulocochlear nerve (eighth cranial nerve)

acupressure
a method of relieving pain or curing illness by pressing on particular points on a person's body with the fingertips or thumbs

acupuncture
a method of relieving pain or curing illness by placing needles into a person's skin at particular points on the body

adaptogens
plants that practitioners of herbal medicine claim can decrease cellular sensitivity to stress

adenosine triphosphate (ATP)
a phosphorylated nucleotide $C_{10}H_{16}N_5O_{13}P_3$ composed of adenosine and three phosphate groups that supplies energy for many biochemical cellular processes by undergoing enzymatic hydrolysis

adrenal glands
either of a pair of complex endocrine organs near the anterior

medial border of the kidney consisting of a mesodermal cortex that produces glucocorticoid, mineralocorticoid, and androgenic hormones and an ectodermal medulla that produces epinephrine and norepinephrine

advent
a coming into being or use

aflatoxin
any of several carcinogenic mycotoxins that are produced especially in stored agricultural crops by molds

air-ionizer
a device that uses high voltage to ionise (electrically charge) air molecules

alkaline
containing an alkali or having the qualities of an alkali

allopathic
relating to or being a system of medicine that aims to combat disease by using remedies (as drugs or surgery) which produce effects that are different from or incompatible with those of the disease being treated

alpha lipoic acid
an antioxidant, and appears to have several roles in the body, including the chelation of metals and extraction of energy from food

amylase
any of a group of enzymes (as amylopsin) that catalyze the hydrolysis of starch and glycogen or their intermediate hydrolysis products

anthropology
the study of human races, origins, societies, and cultures

anti-spasmodic
capable of preventing or relieving spasms or convulsions

antineoplastons
mixtures of various chemicals with theoretic support as natural defense acts against various cancers

apathy
the feeling of not having much emotion or interest

apnea
transient cessation of respiration

arame
an edible Pacific seaweed with broad brown leaves which is used in Japanese cookery

artemisinin
an antimalarial drug $C_{15}H_{22}O_5$ that is a peroxide derivative of sesquiterpene and is obtained from the leaves of a Chinese artemisia (*Artemisia annua*) or made synthetically

arteriosclerosis
a chronic disease characterized by abnormal thickening and hardening of the arterial walls with resulting loss of elasticity

asbestos
a soft gray mineral that does not burn, that was used especially as a building material in the past, and that can cause serious diseases of the lungs when people breathe its dust

Ashwagandha
an Indian herb available in many forms; purported use in inflammation, tumors; has been suggested for use as an antidepressant

assimilate
to learn (something) so that it is fully understood and can be used

astaxanthin
a red carotenoid pigment, $C_{40}H_{52}O_4$, produced by certain bacteria, fungi, and green algae and found in wild salmon, trout, and some crustaceans; used in animal feed to impart color and as an antioxidant

asthma
a chronic lung disorder that is marked by recurring episodes of airway obstruction manifested by labored breathing accompanied especially by wheezing and coughing and by a sense of

constriction in the chest, and that is triggered by hyperreactivity to various stimuli

attention deficit hyperactivity disorder (ADHD)
any of a range of behavioral disorders occurring primarily in children, including such symptoms as poor concentration, hyperactivity, and impulsivity.

autoimmune disease
a disease resulting from a disordered immune reaction in which antibodies are produced that damage components of one's own body

ayurveda
a form of holistic alternative medicine that is the traditional system of medicine of India

bacteriostatic
causing bacteriostasis

bigotry
acts or beliefs characteristic of a bigot

Bilberry
any of several ericaceous shrubs that resemble blueberries but have flowers which arise solitary or in very small clusters from axillary buds

bio-Identical
Identical in molecular structure to a compound made in the body

biodegradable
capable of being slowly destroyed and broken down into very small parts by natural processes, bacteria, etc.

biofeedback
the technique of controlling things in your body (such as heartbeats or brain waves) with your conscious mind

biophotonics
biological applications of photonics, a technology based on the manipulation of photons—the quantum units of light.

biophysics
a branch of science concerned with the application of physical principles and methods to biological problems

bisphenol A (BPA)
an industrial chemical compound $C_{15}H_{16}O_2$ that is a component of several commercially useful types of plastic

brain fog
a usually temporary state of diminished mental capacity marked by inability to concentrate or to think or reason clearly

bromine
a nonmetallic halogen element that is isolated as a deep red corrosive toxic volatile liquid of disagreeable odor

Camu Camu
a fruit from the Amazon, considered a 'superfood' because it contains large amounts of vitamin C

candida
any of a genus of parasitic fungi that resemble yeasts, occur especially in the mouth, vagina, and intestinal tract where they are usually benign but can become pathogenic, and have been grouped with the imperfect fungi but are now often placed with the ascomycetes

carcinogen
a substance that can cause cancer

carotenoid
any of various usually yellow to red pigments found widely in plants and animals and characterized chemically by a long aliphatic polyene chain composed of eight isoprene units

casein
one that is produced when milk is curdled by rennet, is the chief constituent of cheese, and is used in making plastics

catalyze
to bring about the catalysis of (a chemical reaction)

CBC
complete blood count

celiac disease
a chronic hereditary intestinal disorder in which an inability to absorb the gliadin portion of gluten results in the gliadin triggering an immune response that damages the intestinal mucosa

cellulase
an enzyme that hydrolyzes cellulose

chelate
to combine with (a metal) so as to form a chelate ring and is a term used to refer to ways in which heavy metals are removed or detoxed from the body

chia seeds
a plant of the mint family, native to the southwestern U.S. and Mexico, having mostly basal, oblong leaves and small blue flowers: the seeds are used as food and as the source of a beverage

chiropractic
a method of treating people who are sick or in pain by pushing and moving bones in the spine and joints

cholera
a serious disease that causes severe vomiting and diarrhea and that often results in death

chronic obstructive pulmonary disease (COPD)
a chronic lung disease, such as asthma or emphysema, in which breathing becomes slowed or forced

codeine
a drug used to reduce pain

cognitive
of, relating to, or involving conscious mental activities (such as thinking, understanding, learning, and remembering)

Complementary and Alternative Medicine (CAM)
a large and diverse set of systems of diagnosis, treatment, and

prevention based on philosophies and techniques other than those used in conventional Western medicine, often derived from traditions of medical practice used in other (non-Western) cultures

continuous positive airway pressure (CPAP)
a technique of respiratory therapy for individuals breathing with or without mechanical assistance in which airway pressure is maintained above atmospheric pressure throughout the respiratory cycle by pressurization of the ventilatory circuit

cosmic radiation
radiation consisting of cosmic rays.

cosmos
the universe seen as a well-ordered whole

Crohn's disease
a type of inflammatory bowel disease (IBD), resulting in swelling and dysfunction of the intestinal tract.

cruciferous
any of a family (Cruciferae syn. Brassicaceae) of plants including the cabbage, turnip, and mustard

cuvette
a small often transparent laboratory vessel (as a tube)

debilitate
to make (someone or something) weak

deep vein thrombosis (DVT)
a condition marked by the formation of a thrombus within a deep vein (as of the leg or pelvis) that may be asymptomatic or be accompanied by symptoms (as swelling and pain) and that is potentially life threatening if dislodgment of the thrombus results in pulmonary embolism

defibrillator
an electronic device used to defibrillate a heart by applying an electric shock to it

dehydroepiandrosterone (DHEA)
an androgenic ketosteroid $C_{19}H_{28}O_2$ secreted by the adrenal cortex that is an intermediate in the biosynthesis of testosterone

deleterious
harmful often in a subtle or an unexpected way

deoxyribonucleic Acid (DNA)
any of various nucleic acids that are usually the molecular basis of heredity, are constructed of a double helix held together by hydrogen bonds between purine and pyrimidine bases which project inward from two chains containing alternate links of deoxyribose and phosphate, and that in eukaryotes are localized chiefly in cell nuclei

dermatitis
inflammation of the skin.

diethyl toluamide (DEET)
A colorless, oily liquid that is used as an insect repellent

disharmonious
lacking in harmony

dissonance
lack of agreement

distension
the act of distending or the state of being distended especially unduly or abnormally

distort
to change (something) so that it is no longer true or accurate

Druids
Celtic people who, in Europe in ancient times, acted as judges, lawmakers and priests and practiced divination

dulse
any of several coarse red seaweeds (especially *Palmaria palmata*) found especially in northern latitudes and used as a food condiment

duodenitis
inflammation of the duodenum.

E. coli
a straight rod-shaped gram-negative bacterium (Escherichia coli of the family Enterobacteriaceae) that is used in public health as an indicator of fecal pollution (as of water or food) and in medicine and genetics as a research organism and that occurs in various strains that may live as harmless inhabitants of the human lower intestine or may produce a toxin causing intestinal illness

earthing
The act of reconnecting your body to the earth's healthy magnetic field by going barefoot or being out in nature; earthing can also be achieved by earthing sheets and other technology (MRS/PEMF) that creates a field like the earth's life promoting frequencies, thus creating increased oxygen utilization and healthy resonance in the cells

Earthing
the safety device of connecting an electrical system in a building to the earth

echinacea
the dried rhizome, roots, or other part of any of three composite herbs (*Echinacea angustifolia, E. pallida,* and *E. purpurea*) that were formerly listed in the United States Pharmacopeia, that are now used primarily in dietary supplements and herbal remedies, and that are held to stimulate the immune system

electromagnetic
of, relating to, or produced by electromagnetism

electro-smog
radiation originating in a varying electromagnetic field, such as visible light, radio waves, x-rays, and gamma rays

electroencephalograph
an apparatus for detecting and recording brain waves

electro-hypersensitivity
a condition with a wide range of self-reported complaints—e.g.,

oedema, rashes, sleeplessness, mania, depression, heart palpitations and other adverse medical symptoms—purportedly caused by exposure to electromagnetic fields in the forms of computers, telephone base stations, overhead power lines, etc.

electrolyte
any one of various substances in the fluid of your body that control how your body processes waste and absorbs vitamins, minerals, etc.

electromagnetic field (EMF)
an invisible field of electromagnetic radiation on the spectrum of energetic particles that move as quanta (radiowaves, infrared, visible light, UV light and gamma radiation)

electromagnetic pollution
electromagnetic radiation which has a negative effect on the health of living organisms

electromyograph (EMG)
an instrument that converts the electrical activity associated with functioning skeletal muscle into a visual record or into sound and is used to diagnose neuromuscular disorders and in biofeedback training

elucidate
to make (something that is hard to understand) clear or easy to understand

emanate
to come out *from* a source

Emotional Freedom Technique (EFT)
a universal healing tool that can provide impressive results for physical, emotional, and performance issues

environmental illness
a chronic medical condition characterized by symptoms that the affected person attributes to low-level chemical exposure

epidemic
affecting or tending to affect a disproportionately large number of

individuals within a population, community, or region at the same time

epigenetics
the study of heritable changes in gene function that do not involve changes in DNA sequence

epinephrine
a colorless crystalline feebly basic sympathomimetic hormone that is the principal blood-pressure raising hormone secreted by the adrenal medulla and is used medicinally especially as a heart stimulant, a vasoconstrictor in controlling hemorrhages of the skin, and a muscle relaxant in bronchial asthma

Epstein Barr infections
a herpesvirus that is the causative agent of infectious mononucleosis; it is also associated with various types of human cancers

eustress
Moderate or normal psychological stress interpreted as being beneficial for the experiencer

excitotoxin
an excitotoxic agent that can increase heart rate, cortisol and can impact sleep and proper metabolism

far infrared sauna
a type of sauna that uses light to create heat.

fatigue
the state of being very tired

fibromyalgia
a chronic disorder characterized by widespread pain, tenderness, and stiffness of muscles and associated connective tissue structures that is typically accompanied by fatigue, headache, and sleep disturbances

flaxseed
the small seed of flax (especially *Linum usitatissimum*) used especially as a source of oil, as a demulcent and emollient, and as a dietary supplement

folate
A vitamin of the B complex, found especially in leafy green vegetables, liver, and kidney

formaldehyde
a colorless pungent irritating gas CH_2O used chiefly as a disinfectant and preservative and in chemical synthesis

fungicide
an agent that destroys fungi or inhibits their growth

Gaba
an amino acid $C_4H_9NO_2$ that is a neurotransmitter that induces inhibition of postsynaptic neurons

gauss meter
a magnetometer for measuring the intensity of a magnetic field, calibrated in gauss

GDP
Gross Domestic Product.

genetically modified organism (GMO)
an organism whose genetic characteristics have been altered by the insertion of a modified gene or a gene from another organism using the techniques of genetic engineering

geo-engineering
The deliberate large-scale manipulation of an environmental process that affects the earth's climate, in an attempt to counteract the effects of global warming

ghrelin
a 28-amino-acid peptide hormone that is secreted primarily by stomach cells with lesser amounts secreted by other cells (as of the hypothalamus), that is a growth hormone secretagogue, and that has been implicated in the stimulation of fat storage and food intake

giardia lamblia
infection of the intestine with a flagellate protozoan, which causes diarrhea and other symptoms

gingko
a large Chinese tree that has fan-shaped leaves

glioma
a tumor arising from glial cells

glutathione
a peptide $C_{10}H_{17}N_3O_6S$ that contains one amino acid residue each of glutamic acid, cysteine, and glycine, that occurs widely in plant and animal tissues, and that plays an important role in biological oxidation-reduction processes and as a coenzyme, and is known as one of the most important anti-oxidants needed to protect the body from accelerated aging, oxidative stress and physical decline

grounding rod
a metal rod or pipe which is driven into the ground to provide an electrical connection to the earth

herbicide
a chemical used to destroy plants or stop plant growth

high blood pressure (HBP)
abnormally elevated blood pressure especially of the arteries

high-density lipoprotein (HDL)
a lipoprotein of blood plasma that is composed of a high proportion of protein with little triglyceride and cholesterol and that is correlated with reduced risk of atherosclerosis

holy basil
A kind of basil that is venerated by Hindus as a sacred plant

homeopathy
a system for treating illnesses that uses very small amounts of substances that would in larger amounts produce symptoms of the illnesses in healthy people

homeostasis
a relatively stable state of equilibrium or a tendency toward such a state between the different but interdependent elements or groups of elements of an organism, population, or group

homocysteine
an amino acid $C_4H_9NO_2S$ that is produced in animal metabolism by the demethylation of methionine and that appears to be associated with an increased risk of cardiovascular disease when occurring at high levels in the blood

hydrochloric acid
a strong acid that is used especially in scientific experiments and in manufacturing

hydrogenated oil
an oil with trans-fatty acids that has been chemically changed from a room-temperature liquid state into a solid

hypertension
high blood pressure

hyperthyroidism
excessive functional activity of the thyroid gland

hypnotherapy
the use of hypnosis to help people with emotional and psychological problems

hypoallergenic
having little likelihood of causing an allergic response

immunocompromised
having the immune system impaired or weakened (as by drugs or illness)

indigenous
produced, living, or existing naturally in a particular region or environment

insomnia
the condition of not being able to sleep

insulin
a substance that your body makes and uses to turn sugar into energy

intractable
not easily managed, controlled, or solved

jet lag
a tired and unpleasant feeling that you sometimes get when you travel by airplane to a place that is far away (often several time zones)

kale
a type of cabbage that has wrinkled leaves

ketone
any of a class of organic compounds (as acetone) characterized by a carbonyl group attached to two carbon atoms

kirlian photography
a process in which an image is obtained by application of a high-frequency electric field to an object so that it radiates a characteristic pattern of luminescence that is recorded on photographic film

kombu
a laminarian kelp used especially in Japanese cooking as a seasoning in soup stock

kombucha
a gelatinous mass of symbiotic bacteria (as *Acetobacter xylinum*) and yeasts (as of the genera *Brettanomyces* and *Saccharomyces*) grown to produce a fermented beverage held to confer health benefits

lactic acid
a hygroscopic organic acid $C_3H_6O_3$ that is known in three optically isomeric forms: D–lactic acid, L–lactic acid and DL–lactic acid

lectin
any of a group of proteins especially of plants that are not antibodies and do not originate in an immune system but bind specifically to carbohydrate-containing receptors on cell surfaces (as of red blood cells)

libido
instinctual psychic energy that in psychoanalytic theory is derived

from primitive biological urges (as for sexual pleasure or self-preservation) and that is expressed in conscious activity

lipase
any enzyme (as one secreted by the pancreas) that catalyzes the breakdown of fats and lipoproteins usually into fatty acids and glycerol

listeria
a genus of small gram-positive flagellated rod-shaped bacteria that do not form spores, are aerobic or facultatively anaerobic, and have a tendency to grow in chains and that include one (*L. monocytogenes*) causing listeriosis

lutein
an orange xanthophyll $C_{40}H_{56}O_2$ occurring in plants usually with carotenes and chlorophylls and in animal fat, egg yolk, and the corpus luteum

maca
a Peruvian plant whose roots are used as a stimulant

malaria
an acute or chronic disease caused by the presence of sporozoan parasites of the genus *Plasmodium* in the red blood cells, transmitted from an infected to an uninfected individual by the bite of anopheline mosquitoes, and characterized by periodic attacks of chills and fever that coincide with mass destruction of blood cells and the release of toxic substances by the parasite at the end of each reproductive cycle

melatonin
a vertebrate hormone $C_{13}H_{16}N_2O_2$ that is derived from serotonin, is secreted by the pineal gland especially in response to darkness, and has been linked to the regulation of circadian rhythms

metaphysical
of or relating to metaphysics

Methicillin-Resistant Staphylococcus Aureus (MRSA)
any of several strains of a bacterium (*Staphylococcus aureus*) that are resistant to methicillin and related antibiotics (as penicillin)

and may cause usually mild infections of the skin or sometimes more severe infections (as of the blood or lungs) especially in hospitalized or immunocompromised individuals

microcosm
something (such as a place or an event) that is seen as a small version of something much larger

millivolts
one thousandth of a volt

moussaka
a Greek dish of ground meat (such as lamb or beef) and sliced eggplant

Mrem
millirem

mullein
A herbaceous plant of the figwort family with woolly leaves and tall spikes of yellow flowers, native to Eurasia but now widely and commonly distributed

Myers cocktail
a popular approach for treating fibromyalgia syndrome (FMS)—fatigue, pain, a weakened immune system, etc.—among complementary and alternative medicine practitioners

n-acetylcysteine
A mucolytic agent used to prevent liver injury due to acetaminophen toxicity

narcolepsy
a medical condition in which someone suddenly falls into a deep sleep while talking, working, etc.

nattokinase
an enzyme found in natto, a traditional Japanese fermented soybean dish

naturopathy
the treatment of illness by using diet, herbs, exercises, etc., without using standard drugs or surgery

nitric oxide
a colorless poisonous gas NO formed by oxidation of nitrogen or ammonia that is present in the atmosphere and also in mammals where it is synthesized from arginine and oxygen and acts as a vasodilator and as a mediator of cell-to-cell communication

norepinephrine
a monoamine $C_8H_{11}NO_3$ that is a neurotransmitter in postganglionic neurons of the sympathetic nervous system and in some parts of the central nervous system, is a vasopressor hormone of the adrenal medulla, and is a precursor of epinephrine in its major biosynthetic pathway

nori
dried laver seaweed pressed into thin sheets and used especially as a seasoning or as a wrapper for sushi

off-gas
the emission of especially noxious gases (as from a building material)

opiates
a drug (such as morphine or codeine) that is made from opium and that is used to reduce pain or cause sleep

organic
grown or made without the use of artificial chemicals

oscillococcinum
a proprietary homeopathic preparation that comprises a 200c dilution of dissolved Barbary duck livers and hearts

over the counter (OTC)
by ordinary retail purchase, with no need for a prescription or license.

oxidative dtress
physiological stress on the body that is caused by the cumulative damage done by free radicals inadequately neutralized by antioxidants and that is held to be associated with aging

P6/Nei-Kuan
Acupuncture point known as a treatment for nausea and vomiting

palpitations
an abnormally rapid or irregular beating of the heart (as that caused by panic, arrhythmia, or strenuous physical exercise)

pancreatin
a mixture of enzymes from the pancreatic juice

paradigm
a typical example or pattern of something

parasympathetic
of, relating to, being, or acting on the parasympathetic nervous system

peptide
any of various amides that are derived from two or more amino acids by combination of the amino group of one acid with the carboxyl group of another and are usually obtained by partial hydrolysis of proteins

pharmacogenomics (PGX)
the science concerned with ways to compensate for genetic differences in patients which cause varied responses to a single drug

pharmacopeia
a collection or stock of drugs

phosphatidyl serine
a phospholipid found in mammalian cells

phytate
a salt or ester of phytic acid

phytonutrient
a bioactive plant-derived compound (as resveratrol or sulforaphane) associated with positive health effects

phytoplankton
plankton consisting of microscopic plants

pineal gland
a small body that arises from the roof of the third ventricle and

is enclosed by the pia mater and that functions primarily as an endocrine gland that produces melatonin

placebo
a usually pharmacologically inert preparation prescribed more for the mental relief of the patient than for its actual effect on a disorder

polio
an acute infectious virus disease caused by the poliovirus, characterized by fever, motor paralysis, and atrophy of skeletal muscles often with permanent disability and deformity, and marked by inflammation of nerve cells in the ventral horns of the spinal cord

polyphenol
an antioxidant phytochemical (as chlorogenic acid) that tends to prevent or neutralize the damaging effects of free radicals

polysaccharide
a carbohydrate that can be decomposed by hydrolysis into two or more molecules of monosaccharides

Post Traumatic Stress Disorder (PTSD)
a condition of persistent mental and emotional stress occurring as a result of injury or severe psychological shock, typically involving disturbance of sleep and constant vivid recall of the experience, with dulled responses to others and to the outside world

prolozone therapy
an injection technique similar to Prolotherapy that uses ozone; excellent to restore loose ligaments (for more information, www. robynbenson.com)

proteas
any of numerous enzymes that hydrolyze proteins and are classified according to the most prominent functional group (as serine or cysteine) at the active site

psoriasis
a skin disease that causes areas of your skin to become red and rough and to fall off

psychotropic
having an effect on how the mind works

Pulse Electromagnetic Field (PEMF)
a type of electromagnetic therapy in which small electrical currents are intermittently applied to the body

pulse oximeter readings
measurement of the saturation of oxygen in your blood

Qi-Gong
an ancient Chinese healing art involving meditation, controlled breathing, and movement exercises

quintessence
the essence of a thing in its purest and most concentrated form

radiofrequency
any of the electromagnetic wave frequencies that lie in the range extending from below 3 kilohertz to about 300 gigahertz and that include the frequencies used for communications signals (as for radio and television broadcasting and cell-phone and satellite transmissions) or radar signals

Reactive Oxygen Species (ROS)
molecules and ions of oxygen that have an unpaired electron, thus rendering them extremely reactive

reiki
a system of touching with the hands based on the belief that such touching by an experienced practitioner produces beneficial effects by strengthening and normalizing certain vital energy fields held to exist within the body

resonance
a quality that makes something personally meaningful or important to someone

resveratrol
a trihydroxy stilbene derivative $C_{10}H_{12}O_3$ that is found in some plants, fruits, seeds, and grape-derived products (as red wine) and has been linked to a reduced risk of coronary disease and cancer

ribonucleic acid (RNA)
a substance in the cells of plants and animals that helps make proteins

ribose
a pentose $C_5H_{10}O_5$ found especially in the dextrorotatory form as a component of many nucleosides (as adenosine and guanosine) especially in RNA

road rage
anger and aggressive behavior by a driver who is upset by how another person is driving

S-Adenosyl Methionine (SAMe)
S-adenosylmethionine especially when used as a dietary supplement with the intention of relieving depression or arthritic pain and inflammation

saccharomyces
a genus of unicellular yeasts (as a brewer's yeast) of the family Saccharomycetaceae that are distinguished by their sparse or absent mycelium and by their facility in reproducing asexually by budding

salmonella
a genus of aerobic gram-negative rod-shaped nonspore-forming usually motile bacteria of the family Enterobacteriaceae that grow well on artificial media and form acid and gas on many carbohydrates but not on lactose, sucrose, or salicin, that are pathogenic for humans and other warm-blooded animals, and that cause food poisoning, acute gastrointestinal inflammation, typhoid fever, and septicemia

sciatica
pain along the course of a sciatic nerve especially in the back of the thigh caused by compression, inflammation, or reflex mechanisms

Slippery Elm
a North American elm with coarsely textured leaves and rough outer bark; the mucilaginous inner bark of this tree has long been used medicinally

solar flares
a sudden temporary outburst of energy from a small area of the sun's surface

spirulina
a microscopic filamentous aquatic cyanobacterium (genus *Spirulina*, especially *S. platensis* syn. *Arthrospira platensis*) that is sometimes cultivated for use as food especially as a dietary supplement

staph
a group of bacteria that cause many common illnesses (such as skin infections and food poisoning)

statin
any of a group of drugs (as lovastatin and simvastatin) that in-hibit the synthesis of cholesterol and promote the production of LDL-binding receptors in the liver resulting in a usually marked decrease in the level of LDL and a modest increase in the level of HDL circulating in blood plasma

streptococcus
a type of bacteria that causes diseases in people and animals

strontium
a soft silver-white metal that is used in color TV tubes and red fireworks

sudoku
a puzzle in which several numbers are to be filled into a 9x9 grid of squares so that every row, every column, and every 3x3 box contains the numbers 1 through 9

symptomatic
showing that a particular disease is present

tabouli
a salad of Lebanese origin consisting chiefly of cracked wheat, tomatoes, parsley, mint, onions, lemon juice, and olive oil

Tai chi
a Chinese form of exercise that uses very slow and controlled movements

thermography
a technique for detecting and measuring variations in the heat emitted by various regions of the body and transforming them into visible signals that can be recorded photographically (as for diagnosing abnormal or diseased underlying conditions)

Transcendental Meditation (TM)
used for a method of meditating in which you close your eyes and repeatedly think of a simple sound, word, or phrase (called a mantra)

Trigger Point Injection Therapy
a pain therapy that attenuates muscle spasms by locoregional injection of a procaine solution into painful muscles

triglyceride
any of a group of lipids that are esters formed from one molecule of glycerol and three molecules of one or more fatty acids, are widespread in adipose tissue, and commonly circulate in the blood in the form of lipoproteins

triphala
in Ayurveda, a rasayana formula used to enhance youthful energy, strength, and vitality

ulcerative colitis
a nonspecific inflammatory disease of the colon of unknown cause characterized by diarrhea with discharge of mucus and blood, cramping abdominal pain, and inflammation and edema of the mucous membrane with patches of ulceration

ultraviolet blood irradiation
a technique for blood-borne infections by zapping packed RBCs with UV light

umpteenth
very many

vaccine
a substance that is usually injected into a person or animal to protect against a particular disease

varicose veins
an abnormal swelling and tortuosity especially of a superficial vein of the legs

vertigo
a sensation of motion which is associated with various disorders (as of the inner ear) and in which the individual or the individual's surroundings seem to whirl dizzily

virostatic
tending to check the growth of viruses

wakame
an edible brown seaweed used, typically in dried form, in Chinese and Japanese cooking.

walking meditation
a form of meditation in action

warts
a small, hard lump on the skin caused by a virus

wi-fi
used to certify the interoperability of wireless computer networking devices

xenobiotics
a chemical compound (as a drug, pesticide, or carcinogen) that is foreign to a living organism

yoga
a system of exercises for mental and physical health

Index

Numbers

A

C

F

H

M

P

U

V

W

Appendix A

The Healthy Conscious Traveler's Questionnaire

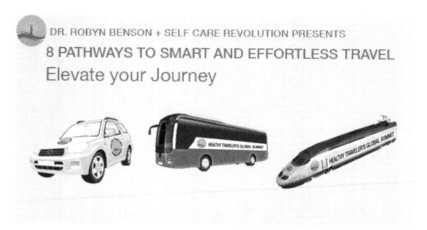

DR. ROBYN BENSON + SELF CARE REVOLUTION PRESENTS

8 PATHWAYS TO SMART AND EFFORTLESS TRAVEL

Elevate your Journey

To find more travel questions from the Healthy Conscious Traveler, go to www.robynbenson.com

Assess Your Healthy Travel IQ!

Are you traveling the healthy way? Assess your knowledge about healthy traveling if you're prepared enough before, during and after your travel. Take the Healthy Conscious Traveler's General Quiz below and increase your travel experience each and every trip.

To take the quiz after every chapter of this book, go to: robynbenson.com

I am on a mission to raise the health bar of global travel. Share and invite your friends, family and loved ones to be part of the Healthy Travel Global Summit at anytime, so they too can be a Healthy and Smart Traveler (http://www.healthytravelerssummit.com/).

Cheers to your healthy travel with each and every trip.

Healthy Conscious Traveler's Quiz

1. What is the name of the high levels of distorting frequencies that emanate from Wi-Fi, cell phones, computers, routers, server rooms, cell towers, cordless phones and plasma screens?

2. Airplanes, cars, buses and trains all emit unhealthy electromagnetic frequencies. True or False?

3. Which is true? Blood oxygen saturation during commercial flights can be 5 to10% lower or higher than normal.

4. What is the name of the hand-held measuring device used to measure harmful electromagnetic frequencies (EMFs)?

5. What is the name of the powerful acupuncture point on the sole of your foot that is strongly rooting, and when activated, helps you return to your connection with the earth?

6. What can be added to water to help rehydrate your body before, during and after travel?

7. What is one of the best ways to avoid high levels of radiation while flying?

8. You can have less radiation exposure when you take your flight at night. True or False?

9. You create inflammation in your body simply by living a stressful life. True or False?

10. What is in our foods, such as vitamins A, C, D and E, which can reduce inflammation response and restore order to our tissues?

11. We can forget about exercise while traveling. True or False?

12. Name an activity that is an excellent way to keep you fit and flexible while traveling.

13. What is a common health problem when traveling, caused by poor hydration and eating too much sugar and foods full of excess sodium, chemicals and preservatives?

14. Most people are dehydrated, even people who drink a lot of water. True or False?

15. What should you do every morning to flush your body of toxins?

16. What chemical released by the plastic containers in the water we're drinking is considered to be an endocrine disrupter and has been linked to a range of health problems?

17. What has a life force that flows naturally and is filled with negative ions and liquid crystals that vibrate in high frequency?

18. Which high-water content vegetable has the exact same mineral composition as bones?

19. How many hours of rest does the National Sleep Foundation recommend?

20. Sleep deprivation causes weight gain or loss?

21. According to Ayurvedic and Chinese medicine, the ideal hours for sleep are between what hours?

22. Alcohol and deep restorative rest can go together. True or False?

23. What is one of the best ways to stimulate melatonin production naturally in your body?

24. Which food helps triple your blood levels of melatonin and gives you healthy omega-3s that can be eaten before you sleep?

25. What do you call being electrically connected to the earth, which helps reset circadian rhythms?

What's your score? You will find out the answers to these questions below and much more as you listen to the 30+ experts on the 10-day Healthy Travelers Global Summit. Visit www.healthy travelerssummit.com.

To take the quiz after every chapter of this book, go to robynben son.com/travel.

Answers

1. Electromagnetic field (EMF)

2. True

3. Lower

4. Gauss Meter

5. Gushing Spring

6. A pinch of salt

7. Sit further away from the window during the day, or if you do have a window seat, close the window cover

8. True

9. True

10. Antioxidants

11. False

12. Yoga

13. Dehydration

14. True

15. Drink two cups of room temperature water with a squeeze of organic lemon

16. Bisphenol-a (BPA)

17. Structured water

18. Celery

19. 7 to 9 hours

20. Gain

21. Between 9 p.m. to 6 a.m.

22. False

23. Sleep in a completely dark room

24. Raw organic walnuts

25. Earthing

Dr. Robyn Benson, D.O.M.
Founder of the Self-Care Revolution
and Santa Fe Soul Center for Optimal Health
Healthy Travelers Summit
505-986-1089

http://santafesoul.com/
http://www.jointheselfcarerevolution.com/
www.healthytravelerssummit.com

Amino Acid Anxiety/Mood and Sugar Cravings/Emotional Eating Questionnaire and How to Boost Serotonin and Gaba Naturally

By Trudy Scott, C.N.

Anxiety/mood issues together with cravings and emotional eating can be a sign of imbalanced brain chemistry and/or nutrient deficiencies.

But they can often be very easily corrected with the use of targeted amino acids, so you can start to feel calm and happy right away. This can give you hope and motivation to figure out other factors (like gluten sensitivity, hormone imbalances, adrenal issues, gut health, etc.) that may be contributing to your anxiety and/or panic attacks and feelings of overwhelm.

Worry and anxiety can be a result of low Gaba and also low serotonin, so you may check off anxiety in both sections. Low Gaba tends to result in a more physical anxiety, while low serotonin tends to result in more anxiety in the head, ruminating thoughts, etc.

Once you address the low brain chemicals, stress eating will just become a non-issue, and you won't be drawn to sugar and carbs. You'll be able to switch off cravings, with no willpower required, and you won't feel deprived. You'll be able to take it or leave it! Really!

Do these questionnaires and see which categories you fall into. And then read on for a few tips for boosting serotonin and Gaba naturally so you can feel calm in your body, relaxed and free from overwhelm, and switch off the obsessive ruminating thinking, and end cravings.

Amino Acid Anxiety/Mood and Sugar Cravings/Emotional Eating Questionnaire

This questionnaire covers all the categories: low serotonin and low Gaba, and low blood sugar, low endorphins and low catecholamines. Many of my anxious clients really resonate with the symptoms of low serotonin (anxiety in the head) and low Gaba (anxiety in the body).

1. Do you have low blood sugar?

- Crave sugar, starch or alcohol any time during the day
- Irritable, shaky, headachy – especially if too long between meals
- Intense cravings for sweets
- Lightheaded if meals are missed
- Eating relieves fatigue
- Agitated, easily upset, nervous

These are all signs of low blood sugar / adrenal fatigue

Stable blood sugar and good adrenals = grounded, no intense sugar cravings

AMAZING AMINO ACID: Glutamine

2. Do you have low Gaba?

- Anxiety and feeling overwhelmed or stressed
- Feeling worried or fearful
- Panic attacks
- Unable to relax or loosen up
- Stiff or tense muscles
- Feeling stressed and burned-out
- Craving carbs, alcohol or drugs for relaxation and calming

These are all signs of low Gaba

Enough Gaba = Relaxed, stress-free

AMAZING AMINO ACID: Gaba

3. Do you have low serotonin?

- Anxiety
- Panic attacks or phobias
- Feeling worried or fearful
- Obsessive thoughts or behaviors
- Perfectionism or being overly controlling
- Irritability
- Anxiety that's worse in winter
- Winter blues or seasonal affective disorder
- Negativity or depression
- Suicidal thoughts
- Excessive self-criticism
- Low self-esteem and poor self-confidence
- PMS or menopausal mood swings
- Sensitivity to hot weather
- Hyperactivity
- Anger or rage
- Digestive issues
-Fibromyalgia, temporomandibular joint syndrome or other pain syndromes
- Difficulty getting to sleep
- Insomnia or disturbed sleep
- Afternoon or evening cravings for carbs, alcohol or drugs

These are all signs of low serotonin

Enough serotonin = Positive, confident, flexible, easy-going

AMAZING AMINO ACID: Tryptophan or 5-HTP

4. Do you have low endorphins?

- Heightened sensitivity to emotional pain
- Heightened sensitivity to physical pain
- Crying or tearing up easily
- Eating to soothe your mood, or comfort eating
- Really, really *loving* certain foods, behaviors, drugs or alcohol
- Craving a reward or numbing treat
- After a tough day at work does eating a pint of ice-cream help? (all that sugar depletes you of key nutrients)

These are all signs of low endorphins

Enough endorphins: Pleasure, joy, feelings of comfort, pain-free

AMAZING AMINO ACID: DPA/D-phenylalanine

5. Do you have low catecholamines?

- Depression and apathy
- Easily bored
- Lack of energy
- Lack of focus
- Lack of drive and low motivation
- Attention deficit disorder
- Procrastination and indecisiveness
- Craving carbs, alcohol, caffeine or drugs for energy

These are all signs of low catecholamines

Enough catecholamines = Energized, upbeat, alert

AMAZING AMINO ACID: Tyrosine

Amino Acid Anxiety/Mood and Sugar Cravings/Emotional Eating Questionnaire and How to Boost Serotonin and Gaba Naturally © 2014 Trudy Scott All Rights Reserved

The above are modifications from questionnaires in *The Antianxiety Food Solution*, which were reprinted (with some modifications) with permission from *The Mood Cure* (2004) by Julia Ross. Nutritional psychologist Julia Ross is one of the greatest pioneers in the field of amino acids, and I had the good fortune to work with her at her clinic, Recovery Systems, for two years.

The Healthy Conscious Traveler's Suitcase

This packing list for the Healthy Conscious Traveler (HCT) will help ensure your travel is stress-free and fun-filled. Please modify it to your specific needs, as you may want to add or delete items that you need or want on your various journeys. Remember to pack in advance. If you are a frequent traveler, always have the basics ready to go, so you can leave at any time. Here's a helpful suggestion: use a list application on your smartphone, or laminate your list and always have it handy. Your list could include:

- Silverware or an eco-friendly equivalent
- Gauss meter, is a tool to measure magnetic fields and EMF pollution (see Chapter 10)
- Empty BPA-free container (for smoothies and water)
- Travel mug for your hot beverages
- Clothing
- Toiletries/First-Aid Kit (See *The Healthy Conscious Traveler's First-Aid Kit*) www.robynbenson.com
- Vitamins, supplements and prescription meds
- Boiron homeopathic medicine for digestive gas called Gasalia
- Earplugs
- Outdoor adventure: hats, gloves, sport or camping equipment, hiking boots
- Bathing suit and PABA-free sun block
- Computer/cord, Thumb drive, iPod, MP3 player, Kindle, tablets, etc.
- Adapter for electrical outlets in country where you are traveling
- Speakers for your iPod, MP3 player, etc.

- Chargers (for computer, iPod, Kindle, etc.)
- Video camera
- Lantern and/or flashlight
- MRS/PEMF device and travel cord (used with an earthing device I always
- travel with)
- Night guard, if you use one (mouth support for the night grinders and more)
- Passport, credit card, insurance card, calling card, etc.
- Binoculars
- Headband (for winter weather and to protect your ears from the draft on flights) Scarves (decorative or for cold weather)
- Extra water (after flying, it's always refreshing to have in your checked-in luggage) when you're feeling tired and dehydrated from flying
- Food (visit Chapter 8 and the *Healthy Conscious Traveler's Food Guide*) Make sure to take your favorite comfort foods and don't forget to take a small container of coconut oil.
- Coffee substitute and/or tea bags
- Stevia
- Wein Products' ozone breathing device (helps to oxygenate the air near your body)
- Sound machine (for the insomniacs and light sleepers, like me)
- Alarm clock, watch
- Running/exercise clothing (shoes, hat, reflective vest, etc.)
- Heart-rate monitor (for die-hard athletes)
- Hair clip, tweezers, nail clipper
- Spiritual /Altar items (deck of blessing cards and other inspirational material)
- Protein shake ingredients and your Magic Bullet or Nutri-Bullet

Acknowledgments

I agree that it takes a village to raise a child (and I have two), but what I also know for sure after writing this book is that it takes partnering with a long list of fabulous, like-minded friends, a supportive family, coaches and people in the book and health world to write a book that matters.

First I want to thank my mom and dad for taking me and my siblings on road trips and camping excursions to the beaches of the Carolinas, Nova Scotia, the Jersey shore and even nearby campgrounds, amusement parks and on other outdoor adventures. Once I got a taste of a small part of this beautiful world, I knew I had to see the rest.

What I loved most about those trips was my father's enthusiasm for driving all night in our green Ford van with purple curtains (that my mother hand made) just so we could wake up to the sound of the ocean waves. Why waste a day in the car, was his thinking, when we could enjoy yet another full day and family time at the beach. I inherited this sense of adventure and appreciation for camping and seeing new places from my wonderful dad, Robert W. Benson.

I want to also thank Elliott Maise for creating a six-week trip across the country when I was only 15 to visit 37 states with a great group of new friends. It was a wildly soul-expansive trip for me. A time to be independent from my birth family and to see this amazing country. On this trip I discovered two of my favorite places on the planet, Santa Fe New Mexico, and the Grand Tetons and other areas of Wyoming.

Next came international travel, which further ignited my travel gene. My first trip out of the country was to St. Croix, V.I. followed by Mexico, Haiti, France, Spain, Portugal, Greece, Italy and England with my dear friends Dee Dee Adams, Diane Sancilio and Amy Stern. Each one of these amazing women, including Margie Howe, Hillary Randolph and my sisters Kristen and Dawn Benson, have been a big part of my life and have challenged me, loved me, and encouraged me to live and fulfill my dreams. And they have each been there for me through my ups and downs in life.

I am grateful to each and every friend I have traveled with, whether for business or spiritual-oriented travel. The list of countries I have explored with Diane Sancilio is long as we share this insatiable desire to learn about the people and the cultures of the world as well its religions and art.

I want to take this moment to acknowledge all the awesome, beautiful people I have met on the road. If you are reading this book now, know that I am talking about you. In some unique way, you have brought insight, laughter, great conversation, and memorable moments and experiences to my life. Thank you!

The person most responsible for encouraging me to write this book is my dear friend Val Alarcon. As we were taking a flight back to Santa Fe from California together, Val said, "Robyn, it is time! Start writing down your thoughts and possible chapters for your travel book. You have been talking about this book for a very long time. Get to it, sister!"

So after years of putting this off, I took out my computer while still on the plane, and instantly all kinds of ideas, chapter headlines, and possible titles for my book started pouring through me. My book had been birthed, and that was about four years ago.

From that day forward, I spent most every Tuesday afternoon for a few months with Val, organizing, researching, and writing my book as we sipped tea, laughed, and ate yummy organic meals prepared by Val. I am forever grateful to her for this jumpstart to *The Healthy Conscious Traveler*.

Around that same time, I enrolled in Christine Kloser's online book writing summit and devoured everything possible on the 'how' of writing a book, because I cared that this book could possibly have a significant impact on people's lives. In addition to Christine, Steve Harrison, Donna Kozik and Ann McIndoo, I am grateful for the life coaching I committed to over the past few years with Lynn Rose, Marcia Weider, Max Simon, Jeffrey Van Dyke, Dan Sullivan, and Babs Smith. I also appreciate being part of JJ Virgin's mastermind group, where I have become friends with many heart-centered health practitioners who are changing the face of health care.

Special thanks to Dr. Mikell Parsons, Dr. Joan Rosenberg, Marcella Vonn Harting, Dave Asprey, Dr. Pedram Shojai, Trudy Scott, Dr. Nalini Chilkov, Dr. Marcelle Pick, Jeffrey Smith, JJ Virgin, Hyla Cass, Susanne Bennett, Dr. Norm Shealy, Barbara and Dr. Larry Dossey, Michael Gelb and all my New Mexico colleagues, including Dr. Christi Alsop and Dr. Glenn Wilcox. Thank you all for your pioneering ways and for your endless encouragement to get this book out in the world.

I want to thank all the people who put endless hours into reading and editing this book: Lynn Cline, Mary Louise Aries, Tom Myers (my clinical assistant extraordinaire), Harmony West (who provided some of her great travel recipes) Venchi Balendez and Michael Jenkins.

I am forever grateful to all my patients who have taught me so much and to the health practitioners, who have been part of my center, Santa Fe Soul Center for Optimal Health. These include my present and past team members Andrea Peralta, Tom Myers, Marian Mills, Kevin Snow, Wesley Kress, Kim Miller, Sudarshan Federation, Felicia Valdez, Kathleen Nagy, and Karen Bomm, who have overseen my center and my practice and been invaluable in creating this book.

Finally, I am blessed by the endless support from my husband Jason Trainor and our two children Harrison and Hannah, for their patience and support of my book-writing journey. They endured the work trips that took me away for many weekends and the countless hours I spent buried in the process of writing this book, allowing me to create my personal *manifesto* on how we can all *travel* healthfully and consciously through everyday life.

About Robyn

One of Robyn Benson's (Doctor of Oriental Medicine) most important life principles is to stretch far beyond her comfort zone. The lessons she's learned as a result, through travel, her medical practice, and her own internal explorations, have changed her life. Now she wants to help you change yours.

Having lost a brother and a good friend by the age of 15, Robyn has long known that she was meant to learn how to live a

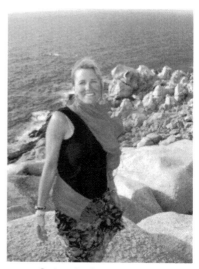

Robyn in Sardinia, Italy

healthy, full and present life, and that she was meant to teach others what she learned. Robyn's knowledge comes from real experience, traveling the world and learning about living well, living long and living life fully.

At home, Robyn spends much of her time researching what she has learned in order to blend the wisdom of her experience with the knowledge of science. She is also able to apply the knowledge gained from her practice at the Santa Fe Soul Center for Optimal Health in Santa Fe, New Mexico.

Robyn founded and built Santa Fe Soul in 2005, with the mission to offer patient's comprehensive and complementary health care. Every single detail of the building was consciously thought out, beginning with a ceremony to bless the land. Santa Fe Soul launched 10 years ago with 25 practitioners who offer 40 different healing modalities, with an emphasis on bridging the best of Eastern and Western medicine.

The mission of this center quickly expanded in 2006 to include a nonprofit called the Santa Fe Soul Foundation. The foundation provides access to holistic and complementary health care through grants and participatory healing opportunities for New Mexico's economically challenged communities, ensuring that Robyn's message is accessible to everyone. In 2013, Robyn was inspired to create a global self-care community called the Self-care Revolution, which continues to grow and impact thousands of people.

"I love taking people through major transformations in their health care," she says. "There's nothing better! And perhaps the most important message of the Self-care Revolution is to help people realize: self-care is a way of life, not an event."

Robyn earned her Bachelor's Degree in Sports Medicine from the University of Virginia and her Master's Degree in Acupuncture and Oriental Medicine at the International Institute of Chinese Medicine. She is board-certified in orthopedic and pediatric acupuncture. With more than two decades of professional experience, she specializes in pain management, women's health and family medicine. In addition to acupuncture, Robyn offers more than a dozen other complementary healing options to her clients, including IV therapies, injections, and cutting-edge energy medicine.

Robyn is married and has two children, Harrison and Hannah. She is a world traveler, public speaker, author, marathon runner and an activist for social change. She has personally brought leading-edge magnetic resonance healing technology to 16 different countries and spoken for four consecutive years at the Tesla Tech Extraordinary Technology Conference (TeslaTech). At the Navigating Your Future conference, she shared the stage with such renowned experts and authors in medicine and healthy living as Jean Houston, Julia Cameron, Michael Gelb and Dr. Hyla Cass.

Robyn maintains her power and passion by taking control of her health and by being an example of a Healthy Conscious Traveler (HCT), no matter where in the world she is. Her greatest driving force now is showing others how to find their own power, no matter where in the world—or in life—they are. She continues to be a learner and endeavors to share her experience and wisdom with everyone.

Made in the USA
San Bernardino, CA
13 October 2015